After Goodbye

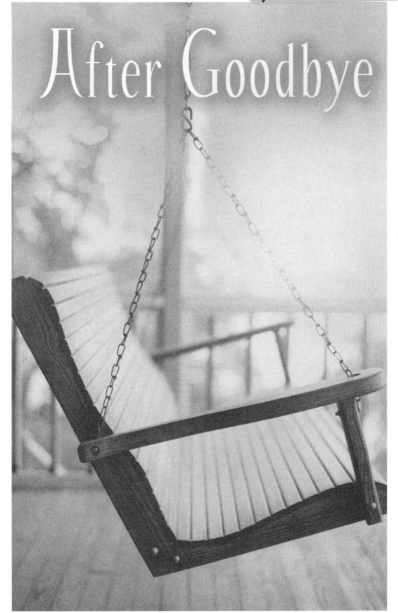

After Goodbye

A Daughter's
Story of
Grief
and
Promise

Lynette Friesen

 SORIN BOOKS Notre Dame, Indiana

www.sorinbooks.com

International Standard Book Number: 1-893732-86-X

Cover and text design by Katherine Robinson Coleman

Printed and bound in the United States of America.

Library of Congress Cataloging-in-Publication Data
Friesen, Lynette.
  After goodbye : a daughter's story of grief and promise / Lynette Friesen.
      p. cm.
   ISBN 1-893732-86-X (pbk.)
   1. Consolation. 2. Bereavement--Religious aspects--Christianity. 3. Grief--Religious aspects--Christianity. 4. Caregivers. 5. Friesen, Lynette. I. Title.

BV4905.3.F75 2005
248.8'66'092--dc22

2004026417

Contents

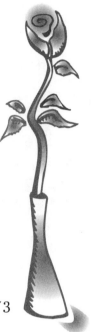

Preface

I invite you, the reader, to reflect on the gift of caring for an elderly parent or loved one. No doubt, many of you will not find time to read this book until after you are no longer the primary caregiver to your parent or loved one. When the right time comes, I hope this book of reflections will help you to ponder your own experiences of caregiving and begin to glean the wonderful gifts you have received in caring for an aging parent. Hopefully, this book is also valuable to those who minister to or are friends of those caring for elderly parents, relatives, or friends.

My mom died peacefully August 1, 1998, at the age of ninety-two. Even though I thought I was prepared for her death, it still came as a surprise. Knowing she no longer had to suffer either physically or emotionally was a relief and brought some peace. But after taking care of her for fourteen years, it was still hard to let her go. During these years since her death, I have reflected over and over again on my own life. I realize so much growth and change has taken place because of what I have learned from my mother, about her and the aging process, about myself and how to love deeply, and about God and my faith.

As I shared my reflections with friends, they encouraged me to put them in a form that could be shared with more people. The experience of caring for Mom, especially during the last four years of her life as she diminished rapidly was extremely stressful. This was a time I needed so much support. Yet the hours of each day were stretched beyond limits and there was no time to seek out the support I so desperately needed. Actually, there wasn't time or energy to even realize my need for support. Only after her death when all her affairs were settled, did I realize the toll it had taken on me physically, mentally, and emotionally. Finally now through reflection and prayer, I have come to realize all the blessings I had during that time and continue to receive because of caring for Mom. In fact, these blessings have made me a more compassionate Pastoral Minister.

The first part of each chapter is the story of Mom's life and mine as it unfolded after Dad's death. The last part of each chapter contains some of the reflections and questions with which I grappled. These questions arose from the particular circumstances of Mom's condition and my unique relationship with her. Each of my siblings experienced things differently because of their own life experiences and unique relationships with Mom. They may share some of my questions, but I know they have their own questions that I can't begin to address. In just that way, the reflection questions I ask may not be yours. You will have questions specific to you, your life experiences, and your unique relationship with your parent and with God.

My hope is that the questions I pose will spark your own questions. I invite you to give yourself the time you need to identify and reflect on them. Your questions may not be answered, but spending time with them can bring a deeper faith and wisdom to your life as well as a greater compassion for others.

Introduction

For almost sixty years Mom lived on top of the hill in Mankato, Minnesota. Seventeen of these years Mom and Dad rented a house on Norton Street at the end of a cul-de-sac. The street was only a block and a half long, and from our porch we could look up the entire length of the street and see Highland Park on the other end. That old house was surrounded on two sides by ravines. For many years there were only two other houses at our end of the street, one to our left just past where the ravine rose up to the street, and the other on the right. Between these houses and the first cross street, most of the land was used as gardens. This was the only home I ever knew until I was fourteen years old.

Mom and Dad bought their first home after my three older siblings, Bob, Lu, and Jim were gone, when my younger sister Pat and I were still living at home. In the mid 1950s a housing development spread along both sides of the street, about one-half block from our house, where formerly there had been gardens. My parents checked into the cost of one of the houses and realized they could afford a down payment with money they had so frugally saved over the years. They were able to get a loan from the owner of the house where we lived, since he was someone Dad had worked for earlier in his life. For years the owner had rented the old house to Mom and Dad for a mere $20.00 per month. Mom and Dad took good care of the house and made many improvements over the years as if it had been their own home. Because of these improvements the owner knew he could sell the house for a profit and was very willing to loan Mom and Dad money at minimal interest. Since the transaction for the new house was complete before it was finished, Mom and Dad had a say in many of the details, and were able to finish the interior as they wanted. In February of 1954 Mom, Dad, Pat and I moved into the new house. Originally the exterior of the house was a pale yellow, but after several years they had it painted light pink. It remained this color until Mom sold the house and moved in April of 1994.

Both Mom and Dad worked and saved every penny they earned to pay the interest and part of the principal each month. Finally when it was all paid for they felt free to enjoy more of life. Dad loved to travel so every summer they went some place. All of their trips around the United States were mainly visits to relatives and seeing the sights in the surrounding areas. By the time Dad died suddenly and unexpectedly in 1984 they had seen the majority of the forty-eight contiguous states plus Alaska. After Dad's death Mom lost her interest in traveling. I was able to drive her to my sister's in Rapid City, South Dakota, a couple of times, and to my sister's in St. Paul for the holidays. Having a full-time job did not allow me time to do more than that.

Mom loved to visit with people, especially her neighbors, when family was not around. She also loved to be outside working on the lawn or in her flower gardens. After Dad was gone she combined the two. She rose relatively early each day and without eating breakfast she began her outside work. As neighbors walked or drove by she took the opportunity to engage them in conversation. This is how she diverted her loneliness.

When I was growing up and my friends would come over, Mom would always stop and talk to them. She loved children and always wanted to hold any baby that she saw, especially her grandchildren and great grandchildren. Her eyes would sparkle as she gave that big smile that so often caught people's attention. It is her smile even up to the day she died that remains in my memory. It is with a smile that I remember her and share our story.

Everyone has, or lives, or is, a story.
In the life review the plot line is
not always clear.
There are many subplots, detours and
wildernesses in each journey.
But connections are made;
we can remember pieces of our lives.

Roy W. Fairchild

1 Dad's Death

Remember the days of old,
consider the years long past;
Ask your father, and he will inform you;
Your elders, and they will tell you.

Deuteronomy 32:7

Monday, March 12 was a bitterly cold day with light snow being whipped around by blustery winds. As part of my pastoral ministry position at the parish in Rochester, Minnesota, I was out making home visits and taking Communion to our homebound parishioners. I returned to the office shortly before noon. Sandie, the parish secretary, asked me to come to her office. As I bounded in to see her, one look told me something was wrong. She asked me to sit down and told me my Dad had died very suddenly that morning. There were no details except that a policeman was with Mom and had done the calling for her. I was immediately plunged into numbness. Very methodically I went back to my office, looked at my calendar for the next week, and made all the calls I needed to cancel my appointments and cover my responsibilities. I then went back to my

apartment, called Mom to let her know I was coming,
packed what I would need, and began the two-hour trip
to Mankato.

It was snowing lightly and as the wind whipped it
around, it froze on the road, making driving treacherous.
Only as I was driving did it begin to sink in that Dad was
gone. I cried and screamed my pain as I drove. This was
the day before Dad's seventy-eighth birthday. I had
planned on going home the following weekend—the
weekend between his birthday and Mom's seventy-
seventh birthday on March 23—to celebrate both of their
birthdays with them.

Mom was watching for me and met me at the kitchen
door. I hugged her as she told me what had happened.
That morning Dad had gotten up as usual and after
breakfast decided to take the pop cans he had collected to
the recycling center. He planned on being home for
lunch. While Dad was gone, Mom was removing the nuts
from the almond bark she made the day before because
Dad was having a hard time chewing the nuts and she
wanted him to be able to enjoy the bark when he got
home. While she was doing this, the front doorbell rang.
There was a policeman who asked to come in and after
they sat down, he informed Mom that Dad had died at
the recycling center. He asked her about family and
whom to call. He called my sister, Lu, in St. Paul and the
parish in Rochester trying to get me. He then called Mom
and Dad's parish in Mankato and one of the Jesuit
Brothers came to be with her. When he arrived the
policeman left. It took me longer than two hours to drive
because of the weather conditions, so Brother was no
longer there when I arrived. Since Mom knew I was
coming she told him she would be okay until I got there.

Some of what happened after Mom told me the details is pretty much of a blur except for one thing—the visit of a young man named Mark. Dad was an easy person to talk to and he had many friends among the young folks all over the city of Mankato. He regularly visited many of the parks and ball fields so he could collect pop cans to recycle. From what Dad told me there were other guys who also tried to collect cans, but many of the young people refused to give their cans to anyone else but Dad saying, "We're saving them for Jake."

Other days when Dad wasn't hunting or fishing he went to a landfill. He looked for anything made of metal, disassembled it and separated the different kinds of metals in preparation for recycling them. At this landfill Dad met a young man named Mark. He was about the same age as some of the grandchildren, none of whom lived close enough for Dad to regularly spend time with them. Dad spent a lot of time with Mark, helping him to know the art of recycling and Mark grew to count on Dad's friendship. Often Dad would take him fishing or hunting. Mark was planning to take Dad and Mom to supper that evening to celebrate Dad's birthday and Mom wanted me to call the landfill and let Mark know what had happened. I could only leave a message for Mark, as he was not there. Within an hour Mark appeared at our kitchen door. I didn't know him at all except from what Dad had told me about him. He was sobbing and in total disbelief. Since I was the one who opened the door, he gave me a hug as he continued to sob, lamenting the loss of his good friend and the fact that he would not have the opportunity to take Dad and Mom out to supper. Mom came to the door as soon as she knew who it was. There was not much she could say to Mark at this point. He wanted to know if he could do anything for us and offered to go to the recycling center and bring Dad's car home. After he left, Mom and I decided we would offer him an opportunity to be involved in Dad's funeral.

My sister Lu arrived a couple hours after I did. The three of us began looking through Mom's address book and making phone calls. I had already called my brother Jim in Boston and my sister Pat in Rapid City. I also called my sister-in-law Dottie in Florida (Bob, my brother had died of cancer in 1973). Both Jim and Pat made immediate plans to come home. Jim and his wife, Marie, would fly in the next morning and Pat, her husband Tim, and their two boys would begin driving yet that night as soon as they could get the car packed. The rest of the evening was spent on the telephone calling extended family. At some time, we must have eaten supper, but everything is such a blur. It was late when we got to bed and I'm not sure if any of us really slept much that night.

By the next morning, my sister Pat and her family arrived. Jim and Marie arrived somewhat later. We went to the funeral home and made all the necessary arrangements. Since Dad was a great collector of black walnuts, and spent his winter days cracking them in the basement when the weather was too harsh for him to do anything outside, we chose a black walnut casket. In recycling metals, he searched most for copper, so we chose a copper vault. At some point during our time at the funeral home, Mom expressed to my sister, Lu, "Now you know what I want when I go!" My sister put it in the back of her mind for future reference.

Sometime before Dad's funeral, Mom wanted to go to the recycling center where Dad died to find out the details of his death. Lu, Pat, and I went with her. We found out that he had just emptied the car of the pop cans and had said something that made both him and the employee laugh. Suddenly he was silent, fell to the ground, and was gone. Dad had often said that when he died, he wanted to go "with his boots on." He did just that. So often he made people laugh by his remarks, and he died laughing. What a wonderful tribute to his sense of humor!

One of my friends, Maggie, also a School Sister of Notre Dame, came to help me plan the wake service and the funeral liturgy. I had done the same for her when her dad died several years previously. She gathered some of our Sisters to help with the music for the wake service Wednesday evening, March 14. Besides Mom and my siblings, most of the grandchildren were there with their spouses and the great grand-children. Extended family who could come were there from both Mom's and Dad's side of the family. Dad was very close to many of his cousins, especially Dave who was a fishing and hunting buddy. Dave had died some years earlier, but his son Earl was there. As Earl and I were talking, Earl put his hand around my shoulder and said, "I bet Dave and Jake are out somewhere fishing right now!"

When I looked at Dad, it really didn't look like him because I remember him so often having a smile or a mischievous grin playing around the corners of his mouth. Then, as I looked at his wispy white hair, I was reminded of how the grandchildren, especially one, liked to play with his hair, forming it into all kinds of shapes. I remember Dad getting ready one time to leave the house with his hair pulled up into two peaks, one on each side of his head. We all laughed as we reminded him to smooth his hair before leaving.

The funeral Mass was Thursday morning, March 15. The grandsons and grandsons-in-law were the pallbearers. Mark, Dad's young friend from the landfill, was an honorary pallbearer. Since Mark did not have a suit, my brother Jim gave him his sport jacket to wear. I know we had picked scripture readings and music we thought were appropriate to Dad. Even though I still have the funeral plans in hard copy, I really don't remember much of anything about the funeral liturgy itself. What I do remember is the wickedly cold day it was when we buried Dad in Calvary Cemetery. As we stood beside his grave I could see Good Counsel, the Motherhouse of my Community of the School Sisters of Notre Dame. I remembered how Dad had been the night watchman there for years. He was always solicitous for the Sisters. He had regular conversations with Sister Alberta who had previously been my Novice Mistress. Here at Calvary he was so close to Good Counsel, and I knew he would continue to guard the Sisters and Good Counsel Hill.

By Friday everyone left to go back home. Since I had made arrangements for my parish responsibilities, I was able to stay with Mom through the weekend. We all had held up quite well before that because we had each other. However, as I sat in the living room with Mom through the weekend, we both had very difficult times. She sat in her chair, and I sat close to her in the chair I always used when I came home. Dad's chair was very visible and very empty. As Mom dozed off, (she was not able to sleep well during the nights) I sat there looking at her. She and Dad had just celebrated their fifty-ninth wedding anniversary February 7. She seemed so small and fragile. I knew the days ahead would be extremely difficult for her. I tried to imagine what her grief was like and I was having a hard time keeping her grief and mine separate.

I did not want to leave her alone, yet I needed to go back to my parish ministry. I also needed to do my own grief work as well as I knew Mom needed to be alone and work through her grief. When I left her Sunday evening, we both cried so hard. I promised I would be back the following Friday as soon as I could get away from the parish. So began my regular trips home every weekend.

As I drove back to Rochester, memories of Dad flooded my mind and heart. He was always there for me with a ready hug. It was Dad who had first recognized my desire to enter the School Sisters of Notre Dame. In fact, when I was a high school senior, Dad and I took a walk one day. He expressed how he just wanted me to be happy in life, and it didn't matter to him what I did or where I went even if I wanted "to become a Sister." I couldn't believe my ears because it was coming from a man who grew up Mennonite, had not known any Sisters other than as my teachers, who was baptized when my oldest brother Bob was baptized, and confirmed when I was confirmed as a sixth grader. I also remember the day I was leaving to enter the Notre Dames and how Dad thought he might never see me again, yet he was willing and ready to let me go even though the sadness was written all over his being. However, it was not a reality that he would never see me again, and his sadness and mine didn't continue for long. I always knew he was very proud of me.

Thoughts came of times when Dad "dropped by" to see me at the schools where I taught when he happened to be passing through or at least close by that town. There was nothing that was too much for Dad to do for me. One time he brought me a second ironing board only because the first one he had brought was not "adjustable" like the second one. When I was preparing for my twenty-fifth jubilee trip to our SSND Generalate in Rome, we had heard that tourists often had their purses stolen when the shoulder strap was cut. Dad brought me a purse with a thick leather strap that was almost impossible to cut.

Other thoughts came of my music ministry at the
parish. When I needed a new guitar and couldn't afford
it, Dad offered me the money so I could get one. I had just
recently paid him back the balance I owed him. I could go
on and on with memories because different people, places
and events are always bringing back memories of who he
was for me. These memories are sacred and keep me
connected to not only who he was for me, but also who
he continues to be for me in my life now.

For Reflection

I had many questions after Dad's death,
questions about life, death, and resurrection. I
wondered what resurrection meant and what
eternal life was like. But since I had to live in the
present without my dad, I wondered how my
mom and I would manage without him. Since I
had grown up believing in the communion of
saints, I also wondered how my relationship
with him would continue.

These are questions that come back to me over
and over again, each time with a new depth.
They cannot be answered with any kind of
certainty, but I need to keep bringing my faith to
the questions and the questions to my faith. I
need to ponder all these things, not in an
intellectual way, but by keeping them in my
heart and learning to live with the paradoxes I
find. One scripture quote I use that helps me on
the journey is this.

At present we see indistinctly, as in a mirror,
  but then face to face.
At present I know partially; then I shall know
  fully, as I am fully known.
So faith, hope, and love remain;
  but the greatest of these is love.

1 Corinthians 13:12–13

It doesn't make any difference how long ago you experienced the death of your parent. What is important is that you spend time with your questions. Wrestle with them and probe them deeply.

◆ What are your questions? Can you name them? Jot them down for yourself.

◆ Who are the people in your life with whom you can share your thoughts and feelings?

◆ What memories do you have of your parent?

◆ In what way are you able to cherish the positive ones and let go of the negative ones?

◆ How is time helping you to understand your parent better?

◆ In what ways has your love for your parent deepened?

◆ Are there scriptures or songs or other tangible things that are meaningful as you ponder your questions?

◆ When have you felt the presence of your deceased parent?

2 Mom's Home

Life is a river
emerging from the springs of birth,
crowned by sacramental blessing:
pulsing through the middle rapids
into pools of mirrored stillness
where is found a clue to meaning.

Wesley F. Stevens

During those weekends with Mom that spring, I really didn't know how to talk about grief with her. Basically I just went home to keep her company and help with the things that Dad had always done. Besides that, there were many things going on in my life at that time. The Friday before he died I had just taken my Master's Thesis to the bindery. Upon returning to Rochester, I needed to pick it up and send a copy to my adviser at Seattle University so I could graduate in May. Sadness closed in on me, realizing that Dad would not be there to enjoy my accomplishment with me. I had also been anticipating my twenty-fifth jubilee trip to Europe. My SSND Community was going to give my classmates and me a trip to Europe. We would spend several weeks

of retreat and pilgrimage at our Generalate in Rome and
some time in Germany visiting the roots of our
Congregation. We were also allowed to travel for two
weeks in whatever part of Europe we chose. Dad had
been anticipating that trip with me by checking out my
plans every time I went home. Now he would not be there
to check out the rest of my plans, nor would he be there
when I returned. He would not hear about all the places
I went or see the pictures I brought back.

At this same time, another situation was unfolding at
the parish in Rochester where I worked. I didn't know
many of the bits and pieces until after I resigned. The
pastor had learned he had cancer of the brain and asked
the Parish Pastoral Council to take over the
responsibilities of the parish until the bishop replaced
him. As a result, the Parish Council was changing my
responsibilities from pastoral ministry and music to
liturgy, an area in which I was not trained. I asked for
two weeks away to discern what to do. I was given two
weeks off with pay, and went to Mankato to stay with a
small group of Notre Dames. After much thought and
prayer I informed the president of the Parish Council that
I was not the one for the job, and would be leaving
in June.

Arrangements were made at the parish to have the
deacon take over the music for me. That relieved a lot of
stress. I could concentrate just on pastoral ministry and
put more time into preparing my résumé and looking for
another position.

The most important thing is that I was free on
weekends to go home and spend the time with Mom. I
was beginning to withdraw emotionally from the parish,
and was drawing closer to her. When I arrived home
Friday evenings, Mom always had supper ready for me. I

don't remember when the change came, but she began sitting in Dad's place at the table, and had me sit in her place. I couldn't help wondering if she started that so that when she was alone, she would not have to look at his empty place at the table, or whether it was just a comfort for her to sit in his place. I never asked her. One of the things she said over and over was that it was no fun to cook now that Dad was gone. She never did eat very much, and it was Dad who ate most of everything she cooked. I was aware that she seemed to enjoy cooking for me when I came home because she didn't have to eat alone.

It was the end of March and there was much lawn work to be done in preparation for summer. The days were getting longer and I could work a little outside after Friday supper. Saturday morning was the time to go grocery shopping with Mom. Then after lunch, I returned to the work in the yard. Often Mom joined me outside. One day as we were raking the leaves, she surprised me with her anger as she said, "I wonder if your Dad knows how much work he left for me to do alone?" I could hear her feelings of abandonment, loneliness, and frustration coming through. I wanted to tell her she was not alone, that I was with her, but it never seemed appropriate to say that because she basically was alone every week five days out of seven. I really didn't know how to respond to her, so I just listened.

Sundays were days of rest for us. After morning Mass and lunch, either we would relax in the living room, often taking a nap, or we would go for a ride in the car. She and Dad had often done that on Sundays. Most of the time we would go out for supper, after which I would head back to Rochester. The Sunday good-byes were always hard. I knew she didn't want to be alone, and I wished I could stay with her.

As I thought of my upcoming twenty-fifth jubilee as a School Sister of Notre Dame, I didn't want to be away from Mom for six weeks. Originally I had planned two weeks of travel with four of my classmates through Germany, Bavaria, Austria and Italy. We would then go on to our Generalate in Rome. My classmates kept pulling me and my sisters kept pushing me to continue with my plans. My sisters assured me they would take good care of Mom while I was gone. Both of them gave me money to help with the expenses for the two weeks of travel through Europe. One day as Mom and I were talking about my trip, she informed me that Dad was also planning to give me some money to help cover the travel costs. Suddenly she stopped, looked at me intently and said, "You know how your Dad loved to travel. He really wanted to go with you—now he will!" We were both flooded with feelings but neither of us could say any more. Looking back on that comment, I realized how her faith in God came through in her statement. Her faith brought me much peace, because I, too, believed that Dad was somehow going to be with me throughout my trip.

The month of May secured for me a new pastoral ministry position in Crystal, a suburb of the Twin Cities, which would begin mid-August. Mom let me use Dad's good car to travel back and forth from Rochester on weekends. Since I had lived in a furnished apartment in Rochester, I had only a few kitchen articles besides my personal belongings. By the first weekend in June I had moved all of these to Mom's basement. I stayed with her until I left for Europe June 14. During these two weeks, Mom decided to get rid of Dad's old car since it was of no use to anyone because we couldn't get it started. She called a junkyard and made arrangements to have the car towed away. When the man came he quickly evaluated the car and decided that the only thing worth something was the hitch. After he paid Mom, it didn't take long for him to hook the car up to the tow truck. Mom and I stood in the driveway and watched it disappear from sight, my arm around her shoulder. Both of us were crying very hard. Mom and Dad had traveled over much of the United States in that car. When they couldn't trust it for extended travel, Dad used it for his short trips hunting, fishing, and recycling. Just thinking of that car brought back many memories, and it was like experiencing Dad's death all over again.

Dad's good car stayed in the driveway. That was the car they used when they traveled together and the one Mom let me use as I moved my things out of Rochester. When she finally needed to get rid of it, my sister bought it for one of her children. Knowing it was still in the family made it easier for her to let it go. She still had her own car that got her wherever she wanted to go.

When the day arrived for me to leave for Europe, two friends of mine offered to drive me to the airport, and took Mom along also. I met the rest of my classmates there. We met my sister from the Twin Cities and visited until it was time to board the plane. It was very hard to leave Mom, but it seemed comforting to both of us to have other friends and family with us when we said good-bye.

While traveling with my classmates and spending time in Rome, I was surprised at how peaceful I was. I know that part of it was feeling that Dad was with me. One of my experiences shortly after Dad's death came back to me poignantly. I was walking early one morning in the Rochester neighborhood where I lived when my foot hit something. I leaned over to pick it up and realized it was a black walnut. I looked all around to find the tree from which it had fallen. There was no black walnut tree anywhere. I thought it was just too dark for me to identify the tree. When I went back in the daylight I could not find any walnut tree either on that street or any of the surrounding streets. This experience spoke to me powerfully of Dad's presence. To this day I still have that black walnut. I missed Dad very much, but somehow, knowing he was "with me" helped me to be peaceful throughout my time away. Because of the peacefulness, I was able to spend a lot of time in quiet prayer while in Rome.

I was concerned about Mom, but I knew my sisters would keep their promise of caring for her in my absence. I also knew that during the summer she would spend a lot of time outside working in her flowers and on the lawn. She would take every opportunity to visit with friends and neighbors.

When I returned from Europe on July 28, I had a couple weeks to spend with Mom before moving on to my new job. It felt like I had been away for months. She seemed to be surviving quite well. As I spent time with Mom she shared with me many of the dreams she had of Dad. At this time they were mainly dreams of loss. Often she would dream that Dad was sitting next to her on the bed. When she put out her hand to touch him, she awoke to find herself alone. These dreams always unnerved her. I was concerned about her and couldn't get in touch with my own grief. The summer had been so peaceful, and as I look back, I wonder if I was in denial about Dad's death, or whether my concerns for Mom overshadowed my own grief. Yet, where had my peace come from?

In mid-August I moved to Crystal. Mom and my sister, Lu, helped me pack up my things and drove me there. I lived in a convent and did not need to take the household things with me. All I needed was my personal belongings. During my time in Crystal, I tried to go home almost every weekend. There were times I could not get there because of bad weather, commitments in the parish, or the need to have some time with friends. Mom got involved with a Grief Support Group in the parish in Mankato. The support group was facilitated by some of our Notre Dame Sisters. Mom was very faithful in going every week. I don't think she was able to talk much about her grief—she hardly ever spoke about her feelings. I knew when she was very sad because she would very easily tear up. But at the support group she heard what others experienced and knew she was not alone.

Mom was still driving her own car and often took friends to Mass with her on weekends when neither Lu nor I could get there. During the week she would drive around Mankato and visit some of her friends. There was one particular friend who came from town regularly to see her. Her next door neighbor, Jean, came over almost every day to check on her. It seemed Mom's need for people was being taken care of.

It was during this time that Mom also learned how to keep a checkbook and pay all her bills that way. She and Dad had always used cash for everything. She was still doing all of her own cooking and cleaning, and only needed help with repairs and taking care of the lawn in the summer, or shoveling snow in winter. Mom was doing very well on her own. She was already in her eighties. At age eighty-one, she had gall bladder surgery and bounced back very quickly. She amazed me!

Mom continued to share her dreams with me when I came home. Little by little instead of dreaming about Dad's presence and then being unnerved by his absence, she began to dream about things they did together when they were young, even before they were married. She dreamt of doing fun things with him, like walking to town from the farm on which they were both employed, going to movies, buying a bag of candy to eat as they walked back home. She shared many things about their life together that I had not known about her and Dad because they never previously talked about those experiences. She began to express more of her feelings than she had ever done before.

I remember a few of my own feelings of grief. There were times, especially if I was alone in the living room, when I looked at Dad's empty chair and felt his absence inside of me. I kept the walnut in my car where I could have it with me wherever I went and that gave me a sense of peace. But most of the time when I was with Mom we were always doing something or going some place. My concern was always for her, rather than thinking about Dad. I think my concern for her postponed my own grief.

After three years at Crystal, I changed positions and moved to a parish in St. Paul. The job had opened up in late spring and by the time I knew I actually had it, most of the other Sisters were settled in their living spaces. My only option was to find an apartment. When I did, I needed all the household things that were stored in Mom's basement. But I also needed to find furniture. My apartment in Rochester had been furnished and this one was not. Parishioners in Crystal helped me find what I needed at garage sales and moving sales. Between second hand things I purchased for less than two hundred dollars, a few things from Mom's basement, and some shelving from my sister, I had all the furniture I needed.

This was the spring of 1987 and Mom realized that the outside of the house really needed to be painted. She thought about hiring someone to do the work. However, after I talked to my sisters and brother, we coordinated our time so we could all be in Mankato together. Between my siblings, the in-laws and Mom's grandchildren, we finished painting her house in two days. At one time, I counted sixteen paintbrushes going all at the same time. Two of the grandsons replaced the patio roof also. It was not much work for anyone, and we all had a wonderful time. After our work each day we had a picnic and either sat in the garage or on the patio. Mom was so grateful, and she often expressed her pride in her family to the neighbors.

Since Mom was still doing very well alone I changed from traveling every weekend to every other weekend. My sister Lu went during the week whenever Mom had doctor, dental, or eye appointments. Things were pretty stable for us and our routines remained the same for a few more years. My sister Pat usually came two or three times a year to spend a week with Mom, at which time both Lu and I went to Mankato so the four of us could spend time together.

After three years at the parish in St. Paul, I changed positions and began work at a parish in Hastings, about twenty-five miles away from where I lived. I continued living in the same apartment in St. Paul and commuting daily. It was during this time Mom slowed down and needed more help. Besides needing me to do the outside work, she also began to need help with the cleaning of the house and cooking. My weekends began to be much more concentrated. I also helped Mom cook and we prepared much more than we needed for our meal together so we could freeze some in small portions for her meals during the week. She was still driving and paying all her bills, but it was just taking her a lot longer to do so.

Things were not always smooth for Mom and myself. We were very much alike—both very strong-willed and stubborn. We both had our ideas on how things needed to be done and when. Since I was taking over more and more of the work, I think I was feeling much more responsible for Mom's care as well as the care of the house and the yard. Most of the time when we disagreed, it was short-lived and it wasn't long before we were back to normal again. However, one Sunday afternoon as I was preparing to go back to the Cities, I was extremely exhausted. I was not looking forward to traveling almost two hours only to have to do my own laundry and cleaning before returning to work on Monday morning. Mom said something to me as we were saying good-bye and it just hit me the wrong way. I objected and we had an argument. It felt terrible because neither of us had time to work it out before I had to leave. I thought about it all the way home, and I know she thought about it that whole time also. When I arrived back at my apartment, I was barely in the door when the phone rang. It was Mom saying she was sorry for making the remark. I, too, said I was sorry and we both burst into tears. Neither of us ever wanted that to happen again.

Mom was about eighty-five years old at this time. She could still move pretty well for that age. One day when hurrying from the kitchen to the bedroom she tripped on an electric cord and took a very nasty fall. As a result she tore the ligaments and tendons in her right shoulder. She was predominantly right-handed and this had serious repercussions for her. She had trouble making out her checks and doing any kind of writing. She wasn't able to drive her car. It was too painful to turn the steering wheel because it did not have power steering. Lu and I decided to have the car equipped with power steering. When Mom's shoulder was healed sufficiently for her to drive the car again, she did so only once. She drove only a little way when she pulled the car over to the side of the road. When I asked her why she did that, she said she did not feel secure enough to drive any more. She was finished. This was the beginning of her being homebound.

I continued to go every other weekend and my sister Lu began coming on the weekends between to make sure Mom got to Sunday Mass. I always drove Mom's car to take her wherever she wanted to go whether that was shopping, to an appointment, or to Mass on Sundays. Sometimes we visited her friends, or took some of them with us to Mass. Even though she didn't drive any more, she enjoyed using her car because she had bought it with her hard-earned money. She had previously bought a second hand car but this was the only new car she had in her entire life. From the time she stopped driving, she kept the car for only about a year and a half. The car was more than twenty years old but was in mint condition with less than 15,000 miles. She knew she really didn't need it since Lu and I could take her wherever she wanted to go in our cars. After I found out the market value for it, one of the grandchildren expressed his desire for it and paid Mom. Mom was pleased he could use it, but she did go through a period of grief because every time she walked into the empty garage she was reminded of her confinement. Mom continued to become more frail and she had less energy and strength.

In 1993 I moved to West St. Paul to live with another Notre Dame Sister, Josie. She was moving from St. Louis to the Twin Cities to begin her doctorate while working in an archdiocesan position. I continued going to Mankato on weekends. More and more of my time was in helping Mom cook good nutritional meals to freeze for the week so she would eat healthy and well-balanced

meals. Because of this, I had less time to do the outside
work, so I engaged a local company to do the lawn
mowing in the summer and snow removal in the winter.
Mom's eyesight was getting dimmer and her writing was
getting shakier. I also noticed that her memory was
beginning to slip sometimes and both Lu and I were
concerned that she would forget to take medication for
her heart condition. We also had concerns about some
other health problems. Lu always accompanied Mom to
the doctor and it seemed the doctor dismissed her
situation because of her age. We were both convinced
that she would be much better if the doctor listened to
her situation and treated her for it. We were tempted to
change doctors, but being from out of town neither of us
knew where to get better care.

With Mom needing more and more help, my
weekends with her were packed so full that I was getting
worn out. It was almost ten years since Dad died. Mom
was approaching eighty-eight years old, and I was also
ten years older than I had been when Dad died. My
energy level was slipping. My ministry kept me busy from
Monday morning to late Friday afternoon, and my
ministry to Mom kept me busy from Friday evening until
Sunday evening. My ability to keep up the pace was
waning and I found myself tired, frustrated, and
sometimes, angry. I had spoken to her at different times
about the need to possibly move closer to Lu and me. I
thought that my suggestions had fallen on deaf ears.
However, I found out later that she had tucked them in
the back of her mind for future reference.

Early in March 1994 a one-bedroom apartment
opened up in my apartment building. I decided to
mention it to Mom when I went home one weekend.
That Saturday was the tenth anniversary of Dad's death.
I prayed to Dad, asking him to help me approach Mom on

the topic. While we were eating supper on Friday evening I told her about the available apartment. I also told her I was getting more and more worn out and I didn't know how much longer I would be able to keep up the pace. Mom didn't say much. Then, Saturday while we were eating supper, she began to ask questions about the apartment and what it would mean for her. I didn't push her because it had to be her own decision. I simply answered all her questions the best I could. On Sunday, I got up early as usual, and was sitting on the living room couch praying when she got up. She came in the living room and sat in her chair across the room from me. She was very quiet and it was obvious she was thinking. Finally she said, "I'm not taking that couch!" I asked her what she meant by that statement and she said, "If I sell my house, I can afford a new one!" She had made her decision. Sunday was March 13, Dad's birthday. I attribute her decision to Dad's intervention. Throughout Sunday we talked more and more about some of the aspects of her moving.

When I returned to St. Paul Sunday evening I immediately called my sister Lu and told her it sounded like Mom was ready to move. Lu went down on Thursday to take Mom to a doctor appointment and then brought her back to St. Paul. She stayed overnight and on Friday the three of us went to look at the apartment. It was available the beginning of April, but since that was much too soon for Mom, the apartment manager said he would hold it until the beginning of May. Mom paid the security deposit to make sure it was held for her.

I was excited about Mom's move. It would be a relief not to have to travel two hours each way every time I went to see her. It would be a welcome relief not to be concerned about the upkeep of a three-bedroom house and all the yard work. A lot less time was needed to clean a one-bedroom apartment. It would be great to have Mom so close where I could drop in on her whenever I had a few moments. Lu could also visit more easily because our apartment building was only two-and-one-half miles from her house. It would be easier to keep track of Mom's clothes that needed to be laundered, I could cook her meals in my own apartment where I had all the ingredients I needed, and she could come to our apartment for some of her meals. Everything seemed so right! I could only see the positive things at this point. I couldn't even imagine or question things that might be hard or difficult. Maybe that was better.

For Reflection

Mom dreamt about Dad a lot and often shared her dreams with me. I had my own dreams about Dad and I wondered why I couldn't share my dreams with her. We often cried together as we talked about Dad but I can't help wondering why we couldn't actually talk about our feelings. I wonder if talking about them would have made things easier for either of us.

There are always those "what if" questions that come back. Until I actually admitted I could not have changed things, I could not let go of some of the guilt feelings. I needed to reflect on all the good things I did do with and for Mom, many of which bring back wonderful memories. It became very important for me to remember the good things.

- What was your relationship with your parent like?

- How has it changed over the years, both before and after his or her death?

- What are your memories of caring for your parent?

- Do you struggle with feeling guilty? About what? Why?

- What are the "what if" questions that keep coming back to you?

- How can you forgive yourself and accept that you did the best you could?

- What do you need to be able to let go of the negative and concentrate on the good memories?

- How has gratitude changed your relationship with your parent?

3 The Move

Thus says the Lord:
"Stand at the crossroads, and look,
and ask for the ancient paths,
where the good way lies;
and walk in it, and find rest for your souls."

Jeremiah 6:16

The decision was made! On Friday, March 18, we informed both my sister Pat in Rapid City and my brother Jim in Boston. The next step was to sell the house. Because Lu was so good at financial matters, she handled that whole thing. One of her high school classmates was a realtor in Mankato so Lu contacted her. We never had to put up a sign in the front yard. The house was close to Mankato State University and was prime real estate. Without even putting the house on the open market, it was sold long before Mom needed to move out at the end of April.

As Lu and I visited Mom throughout the rest of March and April we asked her what she wanted to take with her from the house. We measured her furniture to make sure it would fit into the space in the apartment. We knew she wanted a new couch, but we found out she also needed a smaller table for the dining room. Since the apartment was ready for her, the apartment manager told us we could begin moving things in whenever we wanted. Lu and I took Mom shopping and she picked out her new couch, dining room table and chairs. These were delivered directly to her apartment. On the weekends, Lu and I began to move some of her small things to the apartment piece by piece. I cleaned out things in the basement on weekends, and helped Mom sort out things in the other bedrooms.

There were pieces of furniture that had sentimental value and yet would not fit in Mom's apartment. She and Dad had purchased a bedroom set from the Landkamers in Mankato when she was young and worked for them. It was a double bed, dressing table, and chest of drawers made of black walnut. After Dad died Mom had purchased a twin-size bed and did not want the double bed. She still wanted the dressing table but she offered the bed and chest of drawers to me. I was very happy because it was the only bedroom set I could remember the two of them having from the time I was a child. Mom also had the piano they had purchased from Dad's cousin when I was about ten years old. Mom had planned to give it to my sister Pat but her husband had already bought a piano for her. Since the piano would not fit in Mom's apartment, she asked if I wanted to take it. I did not hesitate at all. Even though Mom first taught me to play on an old piano we had gotten from the neighbors, she had also given me lessons on this new piano. I had spent hundreds of hours at those keys, especially after I started taking lessons from the Sisters. Some of my sheet music was still in the piano bench. Mom also offered me the black walnut dining room table and chairs that had been relegated to the basement to make way for a larger table when they moved into their new house. These pieces of furniture will eventually go to other family members when I no longer need them. It was a comfort to be surrounded by furniture that was so familiar to me.

On Thursday, March 28, my sister, Pat, drove from Rapid City to be with us so we could begin to organize a garage sale with whatever Mom wasn't keeping. She and I worked through Thursday and Friday. On Saturday morning, Lu and Jack came with a moving van. Everything that went with Mom we took out the front door and into the van. Everything else went out the kitchen door into the garage for the sale. We had advertised in the newspapers, so people began coming even before we were ready. We had Mom sit in the living room on the couch she wasn't going to take. Friends and neighbors stopped by and they visited with her there. Her friend Benji came to say "Goodbye."

Benji lived at the end of the cul-de-sac in a large house that had been moved onto the empty lot next to our old house. He was probably about three years old when he first became acquainted with Mom. One thing led to another, and soon Mom was inviting him into the house, giving him any treats she happened to have around, such as animal crackers or candy circus peanuts. He began to come by regularly. From the beginning of Benji's acquaintance with Mom, he could not remember her name so he called her "the pink lady" because she lived in the pink house. Many times, when I was home on weekends, the doorbell rang and there was Benji asking to see "the pink lady." Once in a while he brought a friend or two, but most of the time he was alone. He liked to engage Mom in conversation for as long as fifteen minutes, and then it was time for her to give him some of her treats before he went on his way.

Visiting with friends was a good way to distract Mom from seeing many of her possessions sold. Each thing carried a wealth of memories. As I watched some of her things being sold, especially some she had worked so hard to obtain, sadness began to invade. When it was time for her to leave, I wanted Mom to go to each room and remember some of the things that had happened there and bring some closure for herself. She did go to see the rooms, but the excitement of moving and having us all there made it hard for her to really concentrate on the memories.

Lu's husband Jack and several of their sons-in-law helped move the furniture into the van. Others met them at the apartment in St. Paul to help unload the furniture. Lu drove Mom to St. Paul in her car, while Pat and I stayed until later when we closed up the garage sale for the day. We all met in the Cities that evening for supper. By the time Pat and I arrived, each piece of furniture had been put in its place and her apartment was all ready except for hanging the pictures. She was able to sleep in her own bed that night. Pat stayed with her and slept on the couch (sleeper) so Mom wouldn't be alone.

The next day was Sunday and we went to mass in the morning and spent the rest of the day together. We did a little more in Mom's apartment, but she was pretty well situated already. On Monday, Pat and I went back down to Mankato to open the garage sale again. I cleaned out all the kitchen cupboards while Pat tended the sale. We stayed overnight sleeping on the mattresses that were left. Lu stayed with Mom that night. We did not want her to stay alone until she adjusted to her apartment. Tuesday evening Pat and I returned to the Cities to give ourselves a rest. On Wednesday the two of us returned to Mankato to finish off the sale. By the end of that day everything that was salable was gone. That night there was nothing for us to sleep on so we stayed at a motel. We were back on Thursday morning to finish emptying the house. Josie stayed with Mom that day so Lu and Jack could come to Mankato and help dispose of whatever was left. Anything that was usable went to the Veterans. We finished cleaning the entire house late in the afternoon.

When we closed up the house, I was really having a hard time emotionally. I had my car so I said I needed to do something else yet—can't even remember what it was. I just knew I needed time to say good-bye to all the memories. Pat rode back with Lu and Jack so after we drove off, I turned a corner in a different direction and doubled back to the house again. I needed to bring closure to so many years spent there—memories from my youth, but also from all the years before Dad died when I would go home at least one weekend a month. Then there were the memories of all the weekends I spent with Mom the ten years since Dad's death. I needed to begin the grieving process. I went from room to room, remembering significant things that had happened in each room, thanking that room for its hospitality, blessing it, and saying good-bye. I also went out into the yard where I had spent so much time and did the same there. This was the only neighborhood I had ever known as a child. I was fourteen years old when we moved into this house, and we had moved only one-half block from the where I was born. Mom's moving was severing my last real tie to the entire neighborhood. So I was not only grieving for the house as my home, but also the entire neighborhood and all the memories of friends and neighbors.

As I drove back to the Cities I thought about the house Mom had sold—the only house she and Dad had ever

owned. They had put their life into that house—all the
money they could scrape together and hours of their time
and labor. There were memories of family and friends
who came and stayed. Lu and her husband had come
with their eight children several times each year to visit
when the children were young. Jim had come several
times from Boston with his wife and eight children. Pat
had lived with Mom and Dad each time her husband
went overseas because of his job in the Air Force. Her
two boys, Dan and Jeff, attended the same school we all
attended. They grew up knowing Mom and Dad as
second parent figures. A lot of living took place inside
and outside that house in the thirty years Mom and Dad
lived there together, and also in the ten years Mom lived
there alone. This was not an easy good-bye.

I cried as I left, knowing it could never be the same,
and that I would probably never have an opportunity to
see the inside of the house again. I then drove up to the
cemetery to talk to Dad before leaving Mankato. I think I
was also grieving for Mom because it seemed she was
unable to grieve at this time. I wondered how she would
feel when she realized the finality of it all.

For Reflection

As the years passed, Mom did not talk about
Dad as much as she did at first. I wondered if
she was forgetting him. Possibly she had worked
through the main part of her grief. As she
needed to deal with the loss of her home and
adjust to an apartment, so I needed to deal with
the loss of my childhood home and the last ties
to the neighborhood in which I grew up.

In retrospect, I realize that Mom made her own decisions of when and how to move. As a pastoral minister I meet older persons who feel their children never allowed them to make their own choices. I have also met adult children who struggle with needing to make decisions for their parents because parents try to hang on to a way of life they can no longer sustain. Mom never put any of us in the position of having to make those choices for her. She asked for our help when she needed it but it never felt like she laid a guilt trip on us to force us to do things for her. I am so very grateful!

◆ Who made the major decisions for your parent?

◆ If you had to make the decisions, what are your thoughts and feelings about having to do so?

◆ What are your memories about the home where you grew up?

◆ If you had multiple homes what was it like for you?

◆ If you grew up in only one home, is that home still in the family? If not, what was it like for you when that home was either sold or torn down?

◆ What part did your home and neighborhood play in forming who you are today?

4 The Apartment

Telling the story of our lives is one of the most important activities of the later years. It reminds us that we are still emerging, growing people. It shows us how we have changed and how we have been transformed. . . . [Life review] is . . . a stabilization in the security of the past so that we can go beyond to embrace the future.

Jane Marie Thibault

At first the novelty of the new apartment kept Mom occupied. She liked being close to both Lu and me. Lu came almost daily, at first. I was there daily because she was in my building. She had a balcony off her dining room, and would often go out there and sit. But this just was not home to Mom. After a while she began to grieve for her own home in Mankato. One thing that precipitated that grief was the fact that she could never go outside by herself. I showed her how to go down to the main floor and pick up her mail. But the security door was so heavy, and she was so small and frail that she simply couldn't open the door by herself. She was not able to go out into the yard either. Even though we planted flowers, tomato and green pepper plants on her balcony, she quickly lost interest because they didn't take much care. Without being able to go outside there just wasn't much to occupy her attention. She felt so lost in this huge place and often expressed that she felt like a prisoner because she could no longer go outside by herself. I had not foreseen this kind of a situation, and was very sad for her.

She also loved to visit with people, but she didn't know anyone in the apartment, which only added to her loneliness and isolation. I tried to get her acquainted with a few of the people in the building. I introduced her to Estelle, the woman who lived across the hall from her. Estelle sometimes came over and visited her. Soon Mom began to go over to visit Estelle when she got lonely. In fact, one time I tried to call Mom and she didn't answer. When I went down to her apartment and she wasn't there, I got worried. I happened to hear her voice coming from Estelle's apartment and was glad she was taking the initiative to visit. However, it was only a couple of months before Estelle moved away and Mom's isolation began all over again. Then I introduced Mom to Jane, the woman who lived across the hall from me. Jane went to visit Mom on a weekly basis, and took her outside walking when weather permitted. But it just was not enough.

Mom began to question both Lu and me as to why we took her from her home. Even when I expressed my concern for her and tried to explain that she really made the decision herself, it didn't help. Nothing could quell her grief. I didn't know what to do. I knew she needed to go through her own grief but I didn't know how to help her process it. This was another situation I had not anticipated. As Mom grieved for her home, so did I. Part of my grief was also grieving for her because she was experiencing so many losses.

I continued to cook for her. I usually cooked a big meal in my own apartment, invited Mom up to eat with us, and then put the rest of the food into small microwavable containers. That way she could heat them up in the microwave for herself on the evenings she was by herself. Each morning I went to her apartment and while she ate her breakfast, I prepared her lunch and put it in the refrigerator. When I returned home after work each day, I usually stopped in for a few minutes to see how she was doing. If I had a meeting at the parish I would drop in when I got home. Otherwise, I usually went down after supper to spend a couple of hours with her.

On Saturdays I went to Mom's apartment early in the morning and did her housecleaning. I then gathered her laundry and took it back to my apartment. I did her laundry along with ours and did my cleaning while the laundry was in process. Later in the afternoon, I took all her clean laundry back to her and brought Mom up to my apartment to help her with a shower. Her apartment had only a bathtub and I was afraid she might slip and fall. After her shower, I put up her hair so she would look really nice for Sunday. After supper, I usually went to her apartment to spend time and watch TV with her.

Slowly Mom began to adjust. Even though the apartment building felt very big to her, she was soon able to come up to my apartment on the third floor by herself. On Sundays, Josie and I took her to Mass in the morning, then brought her to our apartment for brunch. She usually stayed the entire day and took her nap on our couch while we were busy reading or preparing supper, etc. If the weather was favorable I took her out for a walk, or a car ride later in the afternoon. She ate supper with us, and after dishes were done and all her meals prepared for her freezer, I went back down to her apartment with her and we watched a couple of her favorite TV shows, such as *I Love Lucy* or *Bewitched*. By the time I got back to my apartment, there was very little time to do anything for myself before needing to go to bed.

At some point, shortly after Mom moved to the apartment, we took her to our doctor who was very respectful and caring. The doctor immediately put her on a diet that cleared up some of her health problems and she enjoyed good health for several months. Sometime during her second year in the apartment Mom ended up in the hospital. Because of her weakness and frailty, she qualified for the services of a home-health aide for a couple hours each day for a few months. This service was such a help to me that when it came to an end, I found and hired a couple of private home health aides. One aide came early in the morning and fixed Mom's breakfast and then her lunch. It relieved me of trying to fix both meals before leaving for work each morning. The aides were also able to help her with some of her personal hygiene.

By the winter of 1995–96, after being in the apartment for more than two years, Mom seemed pretty well adjusted. Having the aides there every day during the week gave her companionship every day. Her ninetieth birthday was coming up on March 23 and Lu and I thought it would be wonderful to have a big celebration for her. Our brother Jim and sister Pat agreed and said they would come for her birthday. I proceeded to make invitations in January and sent them out to everyone Mom had listed in her address book. I knew many of them could not come, especially if they lived at a distance, but I thought the invitations would precipitate her getting a lot of birthday cards.

We made arrangements to use the big party room on first floor of our building that could accommodate a large group. We decided to have an open house from 2 to 4 p.m. on Saturday afternoon. We planned a potluck supper with just family following the open house. We also decided to have a copy of Mom's story for each member of the family.

Before planning for the birthday celebration, I had listened to Mom telling parts of her life story day after day when I was with her, especially when we were eating a meal together. Josie suggested I audiotape her as she spoke. I left the tape recorder on the table and every time she began to tell her story, I clipped the microphone to her collar. I asked her questions to get a more complete story. I can't remember exactly when I started taping, but after almost filling a ninety-minute tape, I transcribed it on the computer. This was probably sometime in January of 1996. Once I had the story typed, I went back and filled in some of the gaps by asking her more questions. The story itself was completed around the end of February.

I made the story into a book. At the beginning was a collage of pictures. There was a picture of her family and Dad's family when each of them were children, a picture of each of them as teenagers, their wedding picture, their fiftieth wedding anniversary picture, and one recent picture of Mom. Her story itself was about twenty pages long. The pages following it were maps of the states where she and Dad grew up and another map of the place they met. The book was completed with a timeline of birth, marriage, and death dates for both her and Dad's family members. We had numerous copies made and Mom autographed each one for family members.

When Pat and Jim arrived a couple of days before her birthday, we decided to go through Mom's old photos and make large posters to place in the party room during the open house. We picked out ones that characterized her life and divided them into five areas: before marriage, early married life, life at 240 Norton Street, life at 218 Norton Street, and the growing family including grandchildren. These we mounted on five large sheets of foam core.

A large general invitation was posted for all the residents of the apartment building. Mom had met many of them at the two previous Christmas parties hosted by the owner of the building and we wanted all to feel welcome.

Lu and I talked about the party for a couple of months before and Mom was anticipating it. Cards arrived from all over the country and added to her anticipation. The day of her birthday finally arrived. She was very excited about her party—probably because she only had one other real birthday party in her life that she could remember. Even though we always celebrated her birthdays, we just never called them parties, or invited friends and extended family to come. She felt so good in the morning and wanted to dress up in some of her nicest clothes. She loved putting on lipstick and perfume, and with a little help she looked wonderful.

In the party room, we had one chair set up in the middle of the room where she could sit and greet people as they came in. As a backdrop, we placed the five posters we had made by the fireplace. They gave friends and relatives a conversation piece as well as a good walk through the history of Mom's life. Several copies of her book were placed on the table so people could read it if they chose. We served cake and punch to everyone who came. The room was always full. One of the grandchildren made a video recording of the people as they came to greet Mom. Besides family and friends, many people from the apartment building came and commented on how they enjoyed the pictures and her book.

After 4 p.m. Lu's adult children brought in the potluck dishes for supper. The two hours of visiting during the open house must have been tiring for Mom, but she didn't show it. She loved to visit and eat with people. We reserved Mom's special treat for supper— angel food cake with strawberries. Before we let her eat some, we all sang "Happy Birthday." She gave us all her great big smile!

The day after the party, before Pat and Jim went back home, we made copies of the video and audiotapes for each of us to keep. Later, we duplicated the five posters for each of us also. These are wonderful keepsakes of Mom and bring back such pleasant memories.

Mom had her own copy of her story that she read over and over again, sometimes several times in one day. I also kept my copy out on the coffee table in my apartment, and after Sunday suppers while Josie and I were doing the dishes, Mom would sit and read her story. She couldn't always remember how it got into a booklet, and asked questions such as "Do you remember when I wrote this? That was some life I had! Have you ever read my story?" As Mom's eyes deteriorated she had a harder time reading her story so I simply substituted a new copy with larger and darker print. Other times I turned on the video of her birthday party. She enjoyed reliving her celebration and identifying the people who greeted her. There was not much I could do with the video of her birthday to help her dimming eyes see better except to have her sit closer to the TV.

Suddenly a few months after her birthday celebration she began to have weak, dizzy spells. We took her to the doctor but nothing specific could be found. I was afraid to leave her alone each day after the aide left at 1 p.m., but didn't know what else I could do since I worked full time. I had the month of July off, which gave me time to be with Mom each afternoon and evening. Lu went on vacation toward the end of July. I figured I could handle everything while she was gone for a week. However, one day Mom had a particularly bad spell and just couldn't come out of it. I got really scared and finally called our doctor, only to find she was on vacation. The doctor I reached, a colleague, said I would need to wait until Mom's doctor returned. I told him she needed medical attention right away. He finally agreed to put Mom in the hospital for observation.

After Mom was in the hospital for several days, Lu returned from vacation. Mom's doctor had not yet returned and she continued to grow weaker. Finally Lu and I insisted they do a CAT scan. Within minutes after they had the results, one of the doctors came to the hospital room to catheterize Mom. They had discovered that her prolapsed uterus was not allowing her to void and everything stored in her bladder was backing up into her kidneys, poisoning her. Within twenty-four hours Mom was feeling much better even though she was very weak. It was also obvious she had experienced some minor strokes because her left hand trembled when she reached for things.

It was fortunate that Mom's doctor returned the following day because, since she had been in the hospital more than a week, the hospital refused to let her stay any longer. The doctor said she would need twenty-four-hour care for a while and insisted we put Mom in a nursing home. It was obvious Mom did not want to go, and I didn't want her in a nursing home either. At first we didn't know what to do.

I spoke to the home-health aides that Mom had before entering the hospital and they were willing to return. We could get some help through Medicare for three months. After many telephone calls we found an aide who could stay overnight and was available later that week. We took Mom back to her apartment and Lu and I took turns staying with Mom the next few nights. With a few more phone calls we filled twenty-four hours of care for Mom each day.

By the end of August an apartment on the third floor opened up next to me. Lu and I spoke for it so Mom could be closer to me. With the help of some of the grandchildren, we moved everything in one day. While we moved her furniture, Josie kept her company in our apartment. Mom slept in her new apartment that evening. Everything was done except the hanging of her pictures. She had moved from a one-bedroom to a two-bedroom apartment. All we needed to do to fill the extra space was to rearrange furniture and get a bed for the second bedroom.

It was obvious Mom was improving day by day and by the end of September she no longer needed twenty-four-hour care. The aide who had stayed through the night still wanted to work, so she began coming on Saturdays and Sundays. Previous to this Lu or I covered the weekends. Now every day was covered from 8 a.m. until

7 p.m. I spent most evenings with her. If I had an evening meeting at work, she would watch TV until I got home.

I loved the evenings I spent with her. They were always relaxing and pleasant. Almost always we had a good laugh, especially as we headed toward the bedroom. She always had a lot of gas, and after sitting all evening, the minute she got up from her chair, she needed to let it go. She tried to wait until she got to the bathroom, but invariably it would escape. The harder she tried to stop it, the funnier it sounded and night after night we ended up laughing all the way to the bedroom. Sometimes she was so bent over with laughter she couldn't walk.

We had our regular ritual. After I helped her undress and get in her nightclothes, she got in bed. Then I handed her one of her rosaries, gave her a big hug and kiss and I tucked her in. Almost always I received a "thank you" for taking care of her along with her big smile.

Even though she seemed to be fine for the evening, I knew it was always possible that something could happen. We purchased a baby monitor and set up the receiver in her bedroom and the speaker in my bedroom. It amazed me how I could hear everything in her apartment, not just in the bedroom. At first I didn't sleep well because I could hear Mom every time she got up to go to the bathroom. When she couldn't sleep, she often prayed the rosary, and not just once! She had three different rosaries by her bed, hers, Dad's, and one given to her by a favorite cousin. If she was still awake after praying one rosary, she would take another and start all over again. She prayed out loud and rattled the beads when she changed rosaries.

Other times she got up and wandered around her rooms. Sometimes she went through her drawers and straightened them or went through things in her desk. One of her favorite things to do was to raid the cookie and candy jars in the kitchen. By the sounds she made, I could always tell where she was and what she was doing. A couple of nights when I knew she was wandering and couldn't hear her, I got worried and went over to see where she was. Invariably I caught her with her hand in one of the jars and she just looked at me with her guilty grin. Eventually I got used to most of the sounds and began to sleep much better. I only needed to know if she was in trouble.

Mornings, after I rose early, prayed, ate breakfast, and washed and dressed for the day, I went over to get Mom up. Before the aide came, while Mom was in the bathroom washing up for the day, I made her bed and chose some clothes for her to wear that day. One of the last things she did after washing was to put on her face cream. She loved to put a dollop on her nose and each cheek before rubbing it in. One day she complained that she was getting as wrinkled as an old prune. I began teasing her about being an old prune and one day she announced to me that even a young prune has wrinkles.

After she was all dressed, I walked her to the dining room where I opened her prayer books for her to the prayers of the day. If I needed to get going before the aide arrived, I kissed her goodbye with a promise to see her later in the day when I returned from work. She prayed until the aide arrived.

Since Mom experienced the weak spells and minor strokes, she was no longer able to go to Mass with us on Sunday mornings. She regularly watched Mass on the local TV station. When the aide left mid-afternoon, I took Communion to her. After we finished the prayers I brought her back to my apartment for supper. One of her weekday aides brought her Communion several times a week. She was always grateful for that gift.

Now that the aides covered eleven hours of each day, including weekends, it was getting more expensive. Since Mom really didn't need constant care during that time, the aides began to help with other tasks. Each one had specific gifts for different jobs. One was an excellent housekeeper, so she did a lot of the cleaning. She was also good at giving Mom a shower. Two others were there for short periods and needed to take care of Mom's breakfast and lunch besides helping her with her personal hygiene each morning. One did some of the cleaning and Mom's laundry. Another was an extremely gentle woman and got Mom outside every day when weather permitted. I still did Mom's grocery shopping and cooking. Having the aides decreased my load of housekeeping chores but it increased other things. I was now supervising their work and doing "payroll" every week.

A problem arose with the weekend aide that I needed to address. She made some very irresponsible choices regarding Mom's care. She knew Mom loved to be out and had asked me if she could take Mom for a ride when the weather was nice. That was fine. However, one day she forgot to give Mom lunch before going out. When she stopped at a grocery store to buy something for Mom to eat, she left Mom alone in a very hot car. Mom had a hard time breathing and was beginning to panic by the time the aide returned to the car. She immediately called 911. All Mom really needed was to get out of the hot car and have a chance to calm down a little. That incident, which could have been avoided, cost Mom $500. Of course, the aide didn't tell me right away.

One evening I went over to spend time with Mom and she wasn't home. It was after dark and I was worried. By the time the aide returned with her, Mom was exhausted. She had taken Mom to a wedding without telling me. When I found out the truth about both incidents, I told the aide she could take Mom out only in the immediate area for no more than a couple of hours a day.

There were a couple of ethical issues I needed to address shortly after this. There were some long-distance calls on Mom's telephone bill and according to the time they were made, this same aide was on duty. She did not inform me she made them. Approximately the same time Mom asked me why this aide was using her shower. I needed to address both issues and found out she had been going down to the swimming pool while Mom was napping. That may have been okay except that she never logged out during that time and we were paying her for all the time she was not caring for Mom. She didn't think there was anything "wrong" with what she did and as we continued to dialogue she said I was being too legalistic. I realized that because of her attitude these kinds of issues might continue to crop up. I didn't want to do that kind of supervision or deal with this kind of behavior so I told her that we could no longer use her services. I had no idea if I would be able to fill her position, but I needed to take Mom's safety and resources into consideration.

Fortunately, one of the other aides who came during the week was willing to work on the weekends also. This particular aide had a wonderful sense of humor. She could get Mom to laugh even when Mom was crabby, which was beginning to happen more often. She spent more time with Mom than any of the other aides. She was good to Mom, and good for her. Mom was also good for her. She confided in Mom and was comforted by Mom's ability to listen and understand.

Even though Mom's mind was pretty sharp most of the time, I found her short-term memory failing more and more. She spoke less and less about Dad and didn't speak of her home in Mankato anymore. Her use of the phone diminished, partly because she didn't have any friends to call here in the Cities, and partly because either the aides or I answered the phone for her. I never called her because it was easier for me to run over to her apartment, and also because I did not want her to fall in hurrying to answer. She had a hard time remembering how old she was and would often ask the question. When she was reminded she was ninety-one she asked, "Why am I still here? None of my family ever got this old." Other times she would remark, "It's heck getting old!"

There were days when she was just very sad, and she didn't know why. I always recognized these times because she walked up to me for a hug and buried her face in my shoulder. All I could do was just hold her. This was easy for me. The hardest days for me were when she was frustrated or crabby. I never knew how to bring her out of it. Usually her mind was sharp at these times and she could really push my buttons. Eventually, I learned that she just needed some alone time, whether that was reading, watching TV, or napping.

One Sunday when she was in the midst of eating supper with us, she suddenly went into one of her frustrated, crabby modes. She pushed my button and I reacted in a negative way. Without finishing her supper, she got up from the table and said she was going back to her own apartment and proceeded to walk out the door. She got confused in the hallway and turned the wrong direction. I kept my eye on her and went to accompany her back to her apartment. She went to her living room and turned on the TV. I asked her if she wanted to finish her supper and she responded negatively so I went back to my apartment and finished my supper. After cleaning up the dishes and putting everything away, I went over to Mom's and found her in a totally different mode. I asked her if she was hungry, and when she responded positively, I heated some of the food I brought with me, and spent a very pleasant rest of the evening with her.

For Reflection

There were difficulties Mom faced in adjusting to the apartment. After a while I realized that when she questioned me about why I took her out of her home, she didn't need a rational answer but rather a chance to talk to someone who would listen to her feelings and understand with compassion.

Slowly I began to realize that the roles of mother and daughter were changing. Even while Mom was still in Mankato, she was in *her* home and I was still her daughter who was helping out. As she diminished in both body and memory, she needed more assurances, encouragement, and affection. It was not a sudden change, but one day I realized this was not the strong, confident Mom I had known earlier in life. I had, in a sense, become her parent. It was hard losing the mothering she had given me. My grief and profound sense of loss went hand-in-hand with learning parenting skills.

I struggled with Mom's shifting moods and behavior, wondering if they were due to the aging process, the minor strokes, her overwhelming sense of loss and grief or some combination of all three. There were times I ranted and raged at God for allowing her to experience such frustration. I was angry with God because it was so hard for me to watch her diminish. It hurt so much to see her suffer. I needed to accept that I could not change what was happening to her; I could not reverse it. I did care for her very well, and she often expressed her gratitude. It is the positive memories I need to keep.

◆ Did you find yourself becoming a parent to your parent?

◆ How did you deal with this responsibility of care?

◆ What were the losses you experienced in this process? How did you grieve them?

◆ How did you deal with your parent repeating the same stories or questions over and over?

◆ How and when did it occur to you that telling the stories was his or her way of reviewing life?

◆ What do you remember of the stories he/she told? What meanings do the stories carry for you now?

◆ What questions did your parent ask that seemed accusatory? How did you deal with them and the emotions they evoked?

◆ What were the care issues you had to address for your parent? How did you deal with them?

◆ How did you deal with the experiences and feelings of your parent's diminishment?

5 Mom's Fall

Very truly, I tell you, when you were younger,
you used to fasten your own belt and go
wherever you wished. But when you grow old,
you will stretch out your hands, and someone
else will fasten a belt around you and take you
where you do not wish to go.

John 21:18

It was almost 10 p.m. on Tuesday, February 3, 1998, when I got home from one of my parish meetings. I had just gone to my bedroom when through the monitor I heard a dull thud and then a blood-curdling scream as Mom cried out in pain. Instantly Josie and I ran over to her apartment. She was in the bathroom, kneeling on the floor, with her hand to her head. She had tripped on her pants, fell forward and hit her forehead on the corner of the door. Josie immediately ran for ice while I helped her up and over to the bed. Even though we applied ice very quickly, the blood-thinning medication she was taking did not allow her blood to clot quickly. After only a few seconds her forehead began to swell. I was scared and quickly called my sister, Lu, whose husband, Jack, was a doctor. They came within minutes. Before they even got there the bump on Mom's forehead was out an inch. I thought maybe Mom would have a headache but she said all that hurt was where she bumped her head. Jack checked the pupils of her eyes for any signs of a concussion, but there weren't any so there was no need to take her to the hospital. She had tripped herself and not fallen because she lost her balance, blacked out, or broken a hip.

We knew Mom shouldn't be alone that night. Lu and I decided to split the night between us. We put up a camp cot at the end of Mom's bed. I stayed with her the first part of the night until 3 a.m. and then Lu took over until the aide came in the morning.

I was so worried about Mom. After Lu and Jack left and Josie went back to our apartment, I sat next to Mom's bed, holding her hand and trying to keep the ice pack on her forehead. She fell asleep numerous times and then would very quickly wake up again. We had given her some pain medication but it just couldn't take away all the pain. During one of her waking moments Mom turned to me and said, "You're not getting any sleep, why don't you go to bed, I'll be okay." I told her I needed to be awake if she needed to get up for the bathroom. She insisted that I needed to at least lie down and not stay beside her. She watched me as I lay down on the cot. She raised herself and said, "That's not much of a bed!" For all the times Mom couldn't track, this night she was amazingly calm and lucid!

I didn't get much sleep that night. She was always so quiet in her movements that I was afraid I might not hear her if she got up. I don't think I got more than thirty minutes of sleep. Lu came right at 3:00 a.m. to relieve me. Even after going back to my own bed (I turned the monitor off) I still didn't get much sleep.

The next day I went to work as usual. Lu took Mom to the doctor and they took a CAT scan of her head. Nothing showed internally, no bleeding, and no damage to the skull. The doctor figured she really didn't hit her head all that hard, comparatively speaking, and that the only reason she had such a bad hematoma was because of the medication. She did tell us that we would probably need someone with Mom twenty-four hours a day because she could have headaches, or be lightheaded and possibly dizzy.

There had been a few hours between the aides' schedules when Mom was alone. Now we were afraid to leave her alone in case her light-headedness or dizziness might cause her to lose her balance and fall again. I spoke to all of Mom's aides to see if they knew of anyone else who would want to work overnight. They all decided to increase their hours to fill in twenty-four hours a day. One of the aides offered to stay most nights. She had no other commitments at that time and needed the extra money. There were some gaps, and that is when Lu and I took turns staying with her. Josie also filled in a few times when we needed someone for a couple hours, especially when I had evening meetings. When we did stay with Mom it was hard to get any sleep because she was up almost every hour.

During these days right after her fall we were faced with difficult decisions about her care. First of all I was exhausted trying to work full time and make sure someone was always with her. I found myself completely worn out. Secondly, one of the aides told me she would be leaving by the end of March because she was getting married and moving out of state. I tried to find another aide who could take her place but just couldn't find anyone. By mid-February I became desperate. Lu and I knew that if I couldn't find anyone, we better start planning to have Mom move into a nursing home. We had no idea if she would continue needing twenty-four hour care, but if she did neither one of us had the energy or time to cover the aide's departure.

Shortly after Mom moved to St. Paul, Lu, Pat, and I had visited some of the nursing homes in the area and had put Mom's name on the list at a couple of places. Within a week after her fall, I called to ask about openings and was told there might be one by the end of February, so I set that as a target date with the director. We also made arrangements at a second private-pay-only nursing home so that if nothing opened up in the preferred nursing home by the end of February, we would have a place to put her until there was an opening. The die was cast. There was no turning back.

The big task now was to prepare Mom for the move. I hated to think about telling her. I was not sure how that would happen. I just prayed for all I was worth, hoping I would find a way. One day when she had a terrible headache, I sat beside her on the couch. As I put my arm around her she put her head on my shoulder. I asked her if she remembered her fall. She said she did not, so I recounted what had happened. I also asked her if she remembered when Grandpa (her Dad lived with us the last five years of his life) had fallen and needed to go to a nursing home. She didn't remember that either so I recounted that story. Slowly I proceeded to tell her that now that she had fallen it looked like she may have to go to a nursing home. She asked, "But where would I go?" As I told her about the home she had many questions at first. Then she fell silent and simply kept her head on my shoulder. I could feel her pain and her fear. I had all I could do to keep from crying. I think she was also holding back the tears. We sat there for a long time as I held her close.

As I experienced Mom through those final weeks in her apartment I began to realize there was a consciousness beyond short-term memory loss. What made me aware of this is that every time she entered the bathroom she said, "I feel like I'm falling." Even though she could not remember her fall, this was a way of remembering. She did not express that in any other room of her apartment. It was hard to determine whether she really could not remember or whether her fear blocked it out. I learned a lot about memory loss even though I couldn't understand it.

Sometimes she could track so well and was very sharp. Even when she repeated herself, she was still able to make sense out of what we said and hold an intelligent conversation. At other times she couldn't track at all. Another thing I learned about short-term memory loss is that the most recent memories go first and slowly the memory recedes further and further. Not only did she forget her home in Mankato, but much of her life with Dad. Then came the times when she confused her brothers and sisters with her sons and daughters. The day had also come when she stopped recounting her story verbally, but she continued reading it over and over again.

In spite of her headaches and dizziness, her sense of humor came through. Just days after her fall the black, blue, green, and purple worked its way down Mom's face and even down her neck. She really looked beat up. Every time she looked in the mirror she asked what happened. One day as she looked in the mirror at her bruises she said she looked like she had a fight with someone. Then she started laughing and said, "I wonder what the other guy looks like!"

She was getting better and by the last week in February she didn't need twenty-four hour care any more. Her headaches and dizziness were decreasing and the night aide did not need to help her to the bathroom anymore. She was getting herself up at night just like she had done before the fall. I so wanted to reverse the decision to put her in the nursing home, but didn't have the energy to do so. Many times I had to force myself to be cheerful when I was with her, even though I was crying inside.

I needed to talk more to her about the nursing home, but wanted to find a time when she was tracking well. The last day of February was Saturday. It was late afternoon the Wednesday before and she was watching one of her favorite TV shows. When the commercial came on I asked her if I could talk to her and she immediately turned off the TV. She was sitting in her favorite chair and I sat on the footstool in front of her, leaning towards her and holding both of her hands. I told her that one of her favorite aides was leaving and I could not find a replacement for her. I really didn't know what to do. I had a full time job and couldn't stay home with her, and Lu had so many commitments she couldn't do it either. Mom amazed me when she said, "Well, aren't there homes for old people like me?" I asked her if she would be willing to go if we could get her into a nursing home.

She did not say yes or no but promptly began to ask about what it might be like and what she could take with her. I told her she could take the chair in which she was sitting. She wanted to know if she could take her drapes and I had to tell her the nursing home already had drapes. She asked about the TV and I told her it was too big and we would get her a smaller one. What really broke my heart was when she asked if she could take her couch. I had to tell her it was too big to fit into the room. She looked so sad and said, "You mean the only thing I'll have to sleep on is my bed?"

For all the years I had known Mom, she rarely lay on her bed for a nap. She always lay on the couch. This couch she had bought less than four years before when she moved to the apartment. It was the nicest couch she had ever owned and she so enjoyed it. Now she had to give it up! I knew she would miss it.

There were only Thursday and Friday left for her to be at home. They were very hard days for her. She moved in and out of awareness that she was leaving her home. The aides experienced her angry moments. She questioned whether her children loved her. They also experienced her sad moments when all she could do was cry and she couldn't even remember why she was feeling so sad.

After her fall and feeling my need for extra sleep I let the aides take over getting her up in the morning so I could sleep later, and let them tuck her in bed at night so I could go to bed earlier. But after making the decision to move her to a nursing home, and when she began to feel better and I felt more rested, I wanted to be with her as much as possible. I began to get her up in the morning and put her to bed at night. I loved helping her get washed up in the morning and watched her put on her face cream. She continued to enjoy putting on lipstick and perfume. I also loved putting her to bed at night because I would always get a good hug and kiss before I left. These were sacred times for both of us and the ones I missed most when I was no longer able to get her up or put her to bed.

By this time, Both Lu and I were so grateful to the aides who so often went out of their way to accommodate Mom's needs and ours. Now that their services came to an end, we wanted to do something for them to express our gratitude. Because part of my job as a pastoral minister was to support caregivers, I had run across a wonderful poem that summed up my own care for Mom and also the care given her by the aides. It was written by one of our parishioners, and I asked her permission to use it. Lu invited the aides to her home for a luncheon and we presented each of them with a matted and framed copy of the poem. I've included it in the Afterword of this book.

For Reflection

The decision to put Mom in a nursing home was extremely difficult for me. I never wanted her to have to go to a nursing home, and I had often told her so. This decision was made without her full knowledge and consent and the pain I felt was excruciating. I know some of the pain was guilt, but I so identified with how Mom would feel. At the apartment she was surrounded by things that were familiar—furniture, drapes and pictures–that she had for years, things I grew up with. I knew there was little she could take with her. She would feel lost and alone in a strange environment with strange people and I already experienced the fear I knew she would feel. It was difficult for me to separate my own feelings from hers. I again ranted and raged at God. I was burning the candle at both ends. Josie, family and friends, supported me but it was just not enough.

I needed to have quality time for myself to gain back some equilibrium. I needed time to just do "nothing" and time to catch up on a lot of lost sleep. I needed time to think, to reflect, to pray, and to rediscover ways to re-create myself. I felt like I was beginning to lose it.

◆ What were your experiences with your failing parent?

◆ Did you need to make decisions for them because they were not capable of doing so? What feelings did you experience?

◆ What kind of support did you have throughout the situation? Was it enough?

◆ How did you feel about God during your care giving? How did you deal with those feelings?

6 The Nursing Home

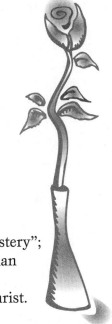

> ... Old age is not only a "natural monastery";
> for many people it is nothing less than
> a sharing
> in the Passion and Resurrection of Christ.
> Nothing less.
> We must honor and cherish,
> support and respect it as such.
>
> *Jane Marie Thibault*

Saturday morning, February 28, came all too soon. The administrator from the nursing home where we wanted Mom to go called Friday to let us know there was an opening. We did not have to put her in the alternate home temporarily. We made arrangements to bring Mom in the late morning so she could eat lunch with the other residents. I felt like I was taking her to prison. I did not sleep all of Friday night. I knew it was going to be a very hard day for both of us.

The only preparations that had been made were having the aides sew names on all the clothes we were taking for her, and marking her name on a few items she could take along. I went to her apartment about 8 a.m. so I could get started packing before she got up. The night aide left for a break but never returned. I think she didn't want to be there for the move. When Mom woke up I helped her get washed up and dressed. I then fixed her breakfast. I tried getting things ready in between, but she wanted me to be with her so I sat down at the table with her. I hadn't had breakfast, but I didn't feel like eating anything.

Lu and Jack came a little later. Then Lu visited with Mom in the living room while Jack and I got things together. I felt so scattered and unorganized, unable to think straight. When we finally had things loaded in their van and my car we got Mom ready to go. She knew we were getting her ready to go somewhere, but she didn't comprehend where. As we put her coat and boots on she was so trusting and docile. She did whatever we asked. I felt like I was betraying her trust. I felt terrible and put in motion my automatic pilot but it wasn't working very well. I was dragging my feet emotionally.

We took Mom down to the van since she was going to ride with Lu and Jack. My car was so stuffed with her things that I couldn't get anyone else in. I got to the nursing home first and found a parking space. I agonized all the way over as I drove alone. Lu and Jack pulled up to the space for unloading. When Jack opened the sliding door and I looked at Mom, I knew she knew, and I knew she felt betrayed. She was sitting there, more or less in a stupor. Lu said that on the way over she had told Mom that she was going to the nursing home. Mom simply couldn't move. When I walked over to her I saw the hurt written all over her face and big tears streaming down her cheeks. I asked her to come with me. She looked at me through her tears and weakly shook her head.

I put my arms around her and cried with her. As I did so I whispered in her ear what I had explained the previous Wednesday—that the main aide was leaving and I couldn't find a replacement for her. She needed care and with my job I couldn't give the kind of care she needed. I couldn't leave her alone day after day but needed to make sure she was taken care of. I just didn't know what else to do. I pleaded with her to please come with me and at least try it. When her foot finally moved towards the door, I knew she would come. She stepped down to the running board and then to the ground with my help. We had her sit in her wheelchair to make it easier for her to get inside, and then entered the handicapped entrance.

Once inside, all the people distracted her. It was lunchtime and they had prepared a place for her in the dining room. Lu stayed with her there while Jack and I set up her room. We lined her dresser drawers before unpacking her clothes, and made the bed with her own linens and blanket. We did as much as we could before she finished lunch. Lu said she seemed to enjoy the company of the other ladies around the table and entered into conversation with them. She didn't eat much because she was too busy talking.

Shortly after lunch Lu and Jack left. I stayed with Mom, talking to her, arranging her room, etc. She was in a double room and it was a real challenge to even find space for any of her things. I had hoped to bring her bed and dresser from home but the nursing home wouldn't allow us to do so. Mom's bed was by the door. In actuality it meant she had no space she could call her own. The space on the left side of her bed was walking space for anyone coming in and out or going to the bathroom. There was barely enough room to put her small chair and little nightstand next to her bed. The space on the right side of her bed belonged to the other person in the room.

I helped Mom get acquainted with where things were in her room. I stayed with her until it was obvious she needed a nap. It was already mid-afternoon. When Mom lay down on the bed I told her I would go home and get some lunch while she napped, since I hadn't had anything to eat all day. I asked her how she was doing. She said, "My heart is pounding. I'll be okay until you get back." I kissed her and told her I would be back in less than two hours. I was hoping Mom could rest while I was gone.

I was back with Mom in about an hour and a half. She was up. I wasn't sure she had ever really slept, but at least she had survived her first hours alone. I accompanied her to supper where she again entered into a lively conversation with the other ladies. She ate well. After supper we went back to her room where I continued to arrange a few things. We turned on the TV, but since there was no cable, we couldn't find any of her favorite old shows. We watched it for a little while and both of us quickly lost interest. For want of something else to do, we just sat and visited.

When she was tired I helped her get ready for bed and tucked her in like I did at home. The nursing home wouldn't allow an electric blanket so I couldn't warm up her bed ahead of time. She had to get into a cold bed. I gave her the rosary and hugged and kissed her good night. I knew she was scared and didn't want me to leave. I didn't want to leave her there either, but she didn't hold me back. I assured her I would be back in the morning. I cried as I left her there thinking about all the feelings of loneliness with which she was dealing. I was also dealing with my own loneliness for her presence in the apartment.

Sunday morning I was up early to shower and got ready to go to the nursing home. The nursing home aides had her up early and she was finished with breakfast by the time I got there. One of the aides told me that she had eaten very well. Breakfast had never been a good meal for her. I'm sure she was distracted by the presence of the other ladies. There was enough time for me to have her put on her face cream, lipstick, and perfume before taking her to the chapel for Mass. Since her room was so far from the chapel, I took her in her wheel chair. We sat almost in the front. As we waited for Mass to begin, Mom leaned over to me and said, "I haven't been to Mass in a long time." She was so happy to be able to attend again. She responded to all the prayers and even tried to sing the songs she knew. Her eyes were getting so bad she could not follow either the Mass prayers or the hymns in the booklet.

After Mass, I visited with Mom until lunchtime. I accompanied her to the dining room and left her to visit with the other ladies while I went home for my own lunch. I promised her I would be back a little later. When I did get back, I again stayed with her most of the afternoon, even while she took her nap. Only after I took her to the dining room for supper did I go back home for my own supper. Later I came back again and stayed the evening until after I had her ready for bed and tucked in for the night. I thought my being there those first couple nights would help her adjust. It also was good for me to not leave her alone so abruptly. Mom was such a trooper!

Monday came and my work schedule started. Every morning that first week I left work so I could be with her for 11 a.m. Mass. I went back to work after I walked her to the dining room. Then, late in the afternoon I returned after work, stayed through the news time and again walked her to the dining room for supper. After I went home and had my supper I returned to visit until it was time to get her ready for bed. She had always loved to watch the Family Channel after supper, but without cable she missed her special shows. This was a real disappointment. The available channels had nothing that interested her. Little by little she stopped using her TV. When she stopped using it, she also lost the knowledge of even how to use the remote control.

The second week Mom was in the nursing home I missed a few mornings Masses with her because of my work schedule. I also had to miss one evening because of a parish meeting. Little by little I reduced the number of times I came until it was only once each day. I wanted to vary my times, but basically it ended up after work. I spent about an hour with her depending on the time I could get away from my office. I gradually cut out the times I went after supper because of the evening parish meetings and my own exhaustion. This was so hard for both Mom and me because putting her to bed was such a sacred ritual for us. It was the time we could really hug each other close and say we loved each other. She often used that time to thank me for taking care of her. Both of us went through a lot of withdrawal. I knew that none of the nursing assistants would spend the amount of time with her either morning or evening that I had spent with her. I cried many times as I tried to let go of that part of her care. I'm sure she may have cried herself to sleep many nights when she missed my care, but she never laid any kind of a guilt trip on me.

One day after I walked her to supper and hugged and kissed her good-bye and she looked at me with tears in her eyes and said, "I miss you." I told her I missed her too. I cried all the way home wishing she could be back in the apartment with everything the way it had been before.

I don't remember the chronological order of events after the first few weeks in the nursing home, but there are certain things that stand out. Mom had been walking with a cane in her apartment but was feeling somewhat unsteady especially after her fall. The nursing home staff was reticent to have her walk with only a cane. Lu and I had asked that her wheelchair be left in a convenient place so we could use it when we there to take her outside. However, the aides wanted to keep her in the wheelchair almost all the time. They did take off the footrests, and one day when I came to see her, I saw her "walking" in her wheelchair. She rolled up to the chapel door, opened it and rolled herself in. Shortly after the door closed behind her she slowly came out again. I remember thinking, "Mom, you are such a survivor!"

It was obvious to us that Mom didn't need to be confined to a wheelchair. She could walk very well with her cane even though she was slow. However, the staff was afraid she might fall and asked us if they could have her evaluated in therapy. We agreed. She passed their test with flying colors but they preferred she use a walker rather than the cane. Lu and I agreed and purchased a walker for her equipped with wheels in the front and "skis" in the back. She seemed to adjust quite well.

Once Mom got used to the walker, there was no stopping her. She went where she wanted, when she wanted. Before long she was walking all over the first floor. She walked more than she ever did in her apartment. I never knew where I'd find her. Sometimes she was in her room, but most often she was sitting in the lounge with the other people. She walked so well with it that one of the aides told me she threatened to give Mom a speeding ticket. She began feeling so confident that many times she walked off without the walker. She didn't have the cane anymore because the staff had asked us to put it away.

Most of the time Mom was fine with being in the nursing home. However, there were those times when she would ask disdainfully, "What is this place?" When I would tell her that it was a nursing home and the reason I needed to bring her there, she would usually go into her own thoughts and not say much. There were times I thought my heart would break when she asked, "Can I come home with you today?" or other times when she asked, "Can I come and eat with you tonight?" I so wanted to bring her home with me, but most of the times when she asked to come were at the last minute or when I had an evening meeting. On the advice of the nursing home staff, Lu and I wanted her to adjust a little more before we took her to either of our homes.

Her ninety-second birthday was March 23 and we planned to bring her to my apartment for lunch. Pat was coming from Rapid City to help us celebrate. The twenty-third fell on Monday, so we chose Saturday, when we didn't have to work. When I got Mom into the apartment, she settled in like she always did. I know she felt at home. There were gifts that she unwrapped, and cards that she read. We took pictures of her with each of us, her daughters. When it was time to take her back to the nursing home, we put on her coat and got her wheelchair. She asked where she was going. When we said we were taking her back home, she said, "If you're taking me home, why are you putting my coat on me?" I know she was thinking of going back to her apartment. When we said she was going back to the nursing home, she had a very hard time. Pat and I took her back. I'm sure she cried inside all the way. Looking into her eyes, it seemed like she was ready to just give up.

When we arrived it was extremely difficult to get her to go in. She resisted, asking over and over, "What is this place?" with disdain in her voice. "Why are you bringing me here?" Once inside we wanted to take her to the dining room for supper. We figured she would be distracted by the other ladies and would forget her time with us. Her feet were like lead and it took forever for her to walk to the dining room. We kept encouraging her but I knew it wasn't only her feet that were heavy—her heart was heavy and so was mine. Once she sat down at table, the other people did not distract her as usual. She was very sad and hurt. There was nothing that Pat or I could say or do that would change things or make her feel better. It was excruciatingly painful to leave her at the nursing home when I really wanted her back home. To her it must have felt like we were not only abandoning her but also betraying her.

Pat and I talked about it on the way home. Both of us were crying, yet feeling so helpless to change the way things were at that point. From that time on, I just couldn't deal with taking Mom home again. I wanted to so often, but I couldn't bear the painful experience of taking her back again. I thought I needed to wait until she was more adjusted to the nursing home when it might possibly be easier. The staff told us that sometimes it takes as long as a year to adjust. As a result, I never brought her home again because she was only in the nursing home for five months before she died.

On Easter Sunday, Lu had invited both Mom and me to her house. I went to Mass with Mom at the nursing home first, then drove her to Lu's. It was not a good day for Mom. She was not feeling well, and couldn't eat dinner. She needed to lie down. We were beginning to realize that Mom was not tracking well that day, and she was not enjoying our company. I ended up taking her back to the nursing home mid afternoon. She was kind of in a daze and didn't say much, except to respond to what I asked her to do. She lay down on the bed. I couldn't help wondering if she was having a hard time because Lu's house was not as familiar as mine was, or if she was dreading the return to the nursing home. I hated to take her back and then leave her there, but I was emotionally shot and knew I couldn't deal with any more grief at that time. I couldn't take away the reality of the aging process for her, or protect her from the losses she was experiencing. All I could do was to try to take care of myself so that our time together was really quality time.

There were some incidents at the nursing home that really disturbed me. I had observed another resident being treated in a very demeaning manner. I reported it, but that didn't seem to change things. I wondered if Mom was treated that way when I was not there. Many of the aides seemed wonderful, but there were some who seemed very unfit for the work that needed to be done.

The only incident we knew of that involved Mom happened one day when Lu came to the nursing home looking for her. Evidently Mom needed to use the facilities and needed some help. Because she was on her way to the dining room, her own bathroom was too far away so the aide took her into the tub room to use the facility there. As Lu walked by, the aide came flying out with Mom in hot pursuit waving her cane at the aide and saying something like, "Who do you think you are to treat me like that? People like you shouldn't be working with people like me. I should report you!" Lu didn't even think of asking Mom what had happened. She just wanted to calm Mom down, knowing the excitement was not good for her heart. Later, Lu didn't want to ask Mom for fear of getting her upset again, and not knowing if Mom would remember the incident. In fact everything had happened so quickly that the aide had disappeared while Lu was trying to calm Mom. Lu didn't have a chance to identify who the aide was. The incident came up at one of the care conferences, but was never pursued because we couldn't identify the aide.

Mom loved to visit with people. However, her short-term memory loss caused her to sometimes ask the same questions or repeat the same story over and over. Evidently there were some residents who got very upset with Mom and were sharp with her. She took it pretty hard and ended up crying. Lu and I were not informed about this. Without warning we received a letter from the nursing home stating that such and such a day they would be moving Mom to the third floor (she had been on first). The letter went on to state that we could contest the move but it basically wouldn't do any good because the decision had been made. I was really upset and asked to know the reason for this move. We had recently had a care conference and nothing had been said to us about a move. They thought it was necessary for Mom's well-being. I had no objections to that, but I did object to the way it was handled. I thought we should have been informed first, then they could have sent the letter because of legal issues. It would have made the whole thing a lot more palatable.

Mom had been in the nursing home only about two months before all this happened. With Mom's move to the third floor, she had no access to the chapel without the elevator, which she could not operate on her own. It was much darker and hotter on the third floor. Lots of equipment for transferring patients was stored in the halls which made it harder for Mom to maneuver her walker. The lounge was filled with wheelchairs, making it difficult for her to navigate there. Most of the people on the third floor were confined to bed or wheelchairs; very few could walk on their own or even visit with her.

The room into which she was moved was directly above her old room, and had the same configuration. Mom was again given the bed by the door. The other person in the room was totally bedridden. Transfer equipment was needed to get her in and out of bed. That equipment needed to be moved completely around Mom's bed to get to the other bed. It was impossible for Mom to have her chair or little table. We originally asked for a private room for Mom but the possibility for that looked pretty bleak. We asked if Mom could have the window side that would give her some space to call her own. It made things easier for the aides to transfer the other lady because they didn't have to move the equipment so far. Our request was granted.

Mom always loved treats and I had kept her supplied with crackers and candy. She had a nice large plastic container for each. When she was on the first floor she could not have them out on her dresser because the lady who shared her room was diabetic. If they were in sight, the other lady would help herself. Because we had to hide them, Mom also forgot they were there. In Mom's new room she could have the crackers and candy on her dresser, so it became a bigger job to keep her supplied.

One day I went to see Mom shortly after she was moved to third floor. I walked up the steps, through the door, and headed for her room. The hallway was so dark I totally missed the fact she was sitting in her wheelchair just inside the hall door. I only got a step or two past her when I heard her call my name. I was surprised she was able to see me in the darkness, but her eyes were probably accustomed to it better than mine were. After this incident, I spoke to the aides and let them know she was not to be in her wheelchair except when she felt too tired to walk. Moving to third floor was like moving her to a different nursing home. She had a whole new set of aides and I had to repeat everything we had asked for with the aides on the first floor.

Each day after work, and every Saturday and Sunday afternoon I spent visiting her. As the weather got warmer I took her outside in her wheelchair whenever possible. If it was a little cool, I bundled her up in her down jacket and hood, put on her boots and wrapped her legs in an afghan. We became familiar with the neighborhood as I wheeled her up and down the streets. As days continued to grow warmer I pushed her longer distances. We watched the trees and bushes blossom out and burst with leaves and flowers. Seeing people planting their flower gardens reminded both of us of the flower gardens she always had around her own home. One day we stopped in front of a house set quite far back from the street. We had spotted a bush by the front door that was covered with purple flowers. A man and his small son were in the yard so I asked what kind of bush it was. Upon telling us it was an azalea bush, the little boy picked one of the flowers and ran over to Mom and handed it to her. She gave him a big smile and thanked him.

The area was full of hills, and I got quite adept at pushing the wheel chair up the hills and holding it back when going down the hills. Sometimes I teased her about needing to get out of the wheelchair and help me push. Several times she actually attempted to get out of the chair and help and we both ended up laughing.

Almost always when we returned to the nursing home, she would ask the question, "What is this place?" When I would explain to her what it was, she would ask, "Why am I here?" "Who brought me here?" I always answered her questions straightforwardly, but it could never satisfy her. As I reflect now, I think her questions had less to do with short-term memory loss than they did with it being so difficult to be there. There were very few people on third floor who were able to visit with her. The people I observed had already "closed down" and seemed unaware that anyone talked to them or cared for them. Her questions made me face the reality almost daily that I could no longer care for her, and it made me very sad.

When weather did not permit me to take Mom outside, there were other things I did with her. I had taken her old picture album that had pictures from when she was a teenager to the nursing home. I asked her about the people in the pictures to get her remembering. Sometimes she would remark that they were really old pictures, but the more recent pictures she simply couldn't identify. Since she no longer read her story to herself because her eyes were getting dimmer, I sometimes read it to her. But little by little even that didn't work because she couldn't concentrate. Other times I took her to the visiting room at the end of the hall where there was a small organ. I played "Name That Tune" with her. She was usually pretty sharp. One day when I played her favorite song "Whispering Hope," she could not think of the title but instead she sang the first line, "Soft as the voice of an angel. . . ." This song came back to me later in a way that spoke to me of her presence.

One of the home health aides gave me a journal she had kept for Mom. Because of Mom's short-term memory loss, she wrote down some of the things they did on a daily basis so Mom could read it. She also wrote down many of the funny experiences they had together, as well as many of Mom's one-liners. One she recorded is the time someone told Mom she was in her "happy golden years" and Mom's quip was "but the gold is all worn off!" In the back of this journal, the aide wrote a note to me after Mom went to the nursing home. I did read it at that time, but I was not really able to appreciate all she said. I will quote some of what she wrote as a fond memory of Mom.

> Hilda was a fun person to be with—we had lots of good times, whether it was walking to the greenhouse, sitting outside, or going to Frank's nursery. Sometimes we just went across the street to the station to get an ice cream cone or a bottle of pop. When I bought a lottery scratch-off, Hilda just shook her head and laughed at me, but she really got excited the day I won over $100. We had long conversations. Sometimes when I felt down, I cried because I missed my son, Stephen. [He died at age eleven of a rare disease.] Hilda listened to me, hugged me and said soothing words. When she had a sad day of missing her husband and other family that died, I would listen, give her a hug and say soothing words.

> We sang songs, did crafts, told jokes and one-liners. When we did silly things we trusted the other never to tell anyone else who might think we were crazy. I could go on and on. I feel so grateful to have had the opportunity to know you and your Mom. Thank you for giving me the chance to be her aide. I sure love her and think the world of you both. I hope one thing for

sure—that when I grow old my son cares for and loves me as much as you have your mother.

During the first couple of months Mom was in the nursing home, Lu and I needed to dispose of her belongings and close the apartment. We left everything alone for the first month. I couldn't bring myself to even begin the process that first month. I had to pass her apartment every time I walked to the laundry or disposed of the garbage. Every time I did, my heart felt so heavy.

The second month I couldn't escape the task. Lu took care of some things and I took care of others. The apartment had to be empty by the thirtieth of April. As I went through her things drawer by drawer, I often cried. As I watched her belongings disappear, I felt I was dismantling her life piece by piece. I agonized over it. As I reflected in an earlier chapter, I believe there is a consciousness beyond the memory loss. I sensed that Mom somehow knew everything that was going on, if not in detail, at least in essence. Slowly she was being stripped of everything that spoke of who she was and what she had done.

In our world "space" and "privacy" equal "wealth." Mom had not only been stripped of her possessions, but also any personal space she could call her own. She literally had nothing anymore, not even privacy. She lost her husband of sixty-plus years, she gave up her home, and she gave up her apartment and all her possessions. She continued to lose her health and her ability to think clearly. She lost most of her eyesight and much of her memory. Mom had become one of the poorest of the poor.

Through the months of June and July, the only times I missed seeing her were the two weeks I was gone for retreat and vacation. During my retreat the first part of July, I chose scripture readings and songs for Mom's funeral. I couldn't explain why, but something compelled me to do so. The third week of July, Josie and I went to Canada with my sister Pat and her husband Tim. When they first came to the Cities, Pat, Tim and I went over to see Mom. What happened was very typical. She was not in her room, so I figured she must be in the lounge. When I went through the door I saw her on the far side of the room. She spotted me immediately and her face moved into a big smile. Her eyes never left my face as I worked my way through and around the wheelchairs to get to her. I helped her through the maze so she could visit with Pat and Tim who were waiting in the hall. She recognized them immediately and enjoyed her time with us.

One week later, after we returned from our vacation, just Pat and I went to see Mom. She was much more tired and very quiet. I guess I didn't think too much about it because she fluctuated from day to day. I never knew if she would be sharp as a tack or find it difficult to track. We took her out for a walk in her wheelchair. Because of the sun, I decided to use her umbrella to shield her. At one point I leaned over and asked her how the umbrella was working. She had a funny grin on her face and said, "Fine, until now. I just can't see where I'm going!" I was totally unaware that when I bent over to ask her I had also tipped the umbrella and it was right in front of her instead of over her. Her sense of humor was still alive and well. When Pat and I left that day, I remember saying to Pat, "I recognize that each day I see her might be the last—I can never be sure I will see her alive tomorrow."

Reflection

I promised to take care of Mom to the end, so
when we had to move her to the nursing home I
felt I was betraying her. I know I made her that
promise in good faith, unaware that I would ever
get so physically and emotionally drained. There
were so many little things regarding Mom's care
that cropped up almost daily at the nursing
home. The aides simply didn't know who Mom
was, nor did they have time to find out. Their
time with each person was minimal, sometimes
hardly sufficient to get the basic needs met. This
was very hard for me to accept because I wanted
the best for my Mother and I felt she was getting
so little. In hindsight, I realize I did the best I
could have done. When the guilty feelings come
I think of what Mom would probably tell me
now. I am sure she would thank me and tell me
not to feel guilty about anything.

- Did you ever make any promises to your parent you
  were not able to keep?

- Did you have to move your parent into a nursing
  home?

- Did you have to dispose of their home and
  possessions?

- What were the feelings this brought on? How have
  you dealt with them?

- How did you feel as your parent continued to
  deteriorate?

- What losses did they sustain?

- What losses did you experience?

7 Mom's Death

There is a time for everything,
and a season for every activity
under heaven:
a time to be born and a time to die,
a time to weep and a time to laugh,
a time to mourn and a time to dance.

Ecclesiastes 3:1–4

Pat and Tim left on Friday. I went to see Mom on Saturday and she seemed to be fine and tracking as usual. Sunday I wanted to go to Mass with her, but she was not feeling well at all. She felt very tired and said she needed to sleep. I went to Mass in the chapel without her. Afterwards I went back to her room, sat in the chair by her bed and held her hand. I stroked her head and just waited for her to wake up. It was getting close to lunch and still she was sleeping. I informed the aides to check on her as I was going home for my lunch. I came back later and she was a little better. I spent the afternoon with her and took her out for a ride around the neighborhood. I commented on things I saw, but she didn't have much to say or even questions to ask as she usually did.

Every day the following week, since I was not working at the parish, I spent quality time with her each afternoon. Each day I either took her for a ride around the neighborhood or into the visiting room to play her songs on the organ. She just seemed unusually withdrawn. I couldn't remember any time she was so quiet for so many days in a row. On Friday when I went to see her, she had been napping and just sat up as I walked in. I went over to the bed and sat down next to her and put my arm around her shoulder. She looked up at me and said, "And who are you?" I answered that I was her daughter. She asked how many daughters she had and I told her three, Lu, Pat and myself. Then she looked up at me with big sad eyes and said, "If you're my daughter, why can't I remember you? What's wrong with me?" She looked very frightened and shuddered.

I asked her if she wanted to go outside. She said yes, so I got her sun hat and sunglasses, had her sit in the wheelchair and took her outside. Because she seemed so extremely tired, and it was rather warm out, we just sat in the shade next to the fountain. I tried to recall stories of her life, or show her pictures to jog her memory, but nothing seemed to work. And to each of my attempts she said, "Why can't I remember? What is wrong with me?" Then she looked at me with fear in her eyes and shuddered.

I was at a loss to say or do anything. When I was silent for a few moments, she turned to me and said, "All I can remember is what's in front of me right now, like this fountain." I had no words because I didn't know how to respond. I simply cooled her arms with water from the fountain, and sat beside her. I stayed until I knew I needed to head for home for supper. I left just enough time to get her back to her room, have her use the facilities and then get her to the dining room. Because of her extreme tiredness, I took her in the wheelchair that evening. I alerted the aides so they would be aware of it. As I said good-bye to her there in the dining room she asked when she would see me again. I said I would be back tomorrow afternoon. She didn't say anything else, but looked at me with sadness very evident in her eyes and gave one last shudder before I kissed her. That was the last time I saw her alive.

Saturday, August 1, I planned to go to see Mom in the early afternoon. I had to do some shopping first in order to refill all of her jars of treats. She had cleaned them out. I got behind as I tried to finish all her laundry and get everything either folded or ironed before taking it back to her. As a result, instead of getting to the nursing home around 1:00, I signed in at 3:15 p.m.

When I went to her room it was very dark—the aides had drawn the drapes again. I had asked numerous times to have the drapes left open during the day because the darkness only confused the days and nights for her. She had a north window and the sun never shone directly into her room anyway. I could see she was lying on the bed as she always did for her nap. After I drew the drapes I bent over to kiss her. The minute I looked at her I knew she was gone. I felt her arms and they were cool, but there was a breeze coming in the window. I felt under her neck and could still feel her warmth. Her eyes were shut and I knew she had just breathed her last within moments before I walked in. I kissed her—a goodbye kiss—and stayed with her for some time talking to her and saying all my good-byes. Even though I knew she would go sometime, I was not prepared to deal with the overwhelming sense of loss.

I slowly shifted into automatic pilot. Eventually I went down to the nurses' station and informed them that Mom was gone. Then I called Lu. Fortunately she was home and answered right away. When I told her Mom was gone, she and Jack came right over. While I waited for them I went back to Mom. I needed to touch her and stroke her head and cheeks. The aides came in one by one or two by two to see for themselves. By the time Lu and Jack came, Mom's eyes were beginning to open, as well as her mouth. I felt her spirit had still been with her when I found her and she heard all I needed to say to her. It was such a gift to have that opportunity! But it was so hard to know I would never be able to experience her coming in for a hug as she used to do. Nor would I see the sparkle that was always in her eyes when she saw me coming or hear her laugh when she said something humorous. Everything felt so final.

None of the nursing assistants could believe she was gone. The one who had gotten her up in the morning said her sense of humor was in fine shape and they had a good laugh before going to breakfast. They did notice that she seemed especially tired and somewhat agitated. When she went for lunch they took her in the wheelchair because she didn't want to walk. She didn't eat much either. They brought Mom to her room and had her lie down for a nap. Because she was restless, they checked on her periodically and were aware she still hadn't slept by 2:30 p.m. Shortly after that she seemed to quiet down. She looked very peaceful as if she had just fallen asleep.

Lu and I went about the tasks we needed to do. From the nursing home we called Mom's doctor to inform her and ask her to prepare a death certificate. We called the funeral home in Mankato where arrangements had already been made. Since they could not get her body that day, they asked us to choose a funeral home in St. Paul that could pick up her body, prepare it for burial until they could pick it up the next day. We also made plans to meet the funeral director in Mankato on Sunday afternoon.

Lu came to my apartment where we spent the whole evening calling friends and relatives and informing them of Mom's death. First we called Jim and Pat. I called Josie, who was in St. Louis visiting her mother. We also called Mom's parish in Mankato and tentatively set the funeral for Wednesday, August 5, and asked to meet with one of the priests Sunday after we finished at the funeral home. Lu and I took turns calling everyone in Mom's address book, and we were able to give them the day for the funeral so they could make travel plans if they could come. Lu didn't leave until late that evening—I have no recollection how late. I know neither of us ate supper. I knew I needed to sleep, but sleep just didn't come. All night my thoughts were of Mom lying on the bed. It seemed she had a peaceful death, and that she had just slipped away. There were no signs of struggle. For this I was grateful, but I couldn't get the image of her out of my mind.

The next morning, Pat's and Josie's planes were due one half-hour apart. After meeting one, it was time to meet the other. We barely had time to go back to the apartment and unload the suitcases before we had to take off for Mankato. The funeral home was first. We couldn't have had a more understanding funeral director. She was wonderful. She was very pastoral, and still kept us on task. One of my ministries in the parish where I worked was to meet with families and help them prepare the funeral liturgy for their loved one, so I appreciated the wonderful ministry we received. It didn't take us long to pick a casket and vault since Lu remembered that Mom said she wanted the same as we had gotten for Dad.

After we were finished at the funeral home, we went to the church to plan the funeral liturgy with one of the priests at the parish. When I planned Mom's funeral during my retreat the previous month, I had narrowed down the Scripture readings and music selections to just a few, so it didn't take long to finalize those. What took the longest was deciding how we would involve family members in the liturgy. I offered to print up a worship aid on the computer at home and have it print-ready when we returned to the mortuary in Mankato on Tuesday afternoon.

Initially, I had planned on spending the weekend at our SSND motherhouse in Mankato because we were having our All-Province Days. Lu and Jack had gone to early Mass that morning, so they drove back to St. Paul after we were finished at the parish. Pat, Josie, and I didn't have an opportunity to attend Sunday Mass, so I suggested we go up to our Notre Dame motherhouse on Good Counsel Hill. There was a 4 p.m. Liturgy. We got there a little late, and found places in the back pews of the chapel. I had called in to the motherhouse on Saturday with news of her death, and it had been announced to the whole community. When people saw me go up for Communion, many of them made it a point to come to me right after Mass. Since Pat looks so much like me, they recognized her as my sister and also greeted her. We stayed for supper. Many who didn't see us in chapel saw us at supper and came to greet us. I felt so supported by all the sisters.

On monday morning, we all met at the nursing home to clean out Mom's belongings. I was so glad we were together because it made the task a little easier. She had so few possessions that we were finished long before noon. Some of the nursing assistants came in at different times as we were packing things up. Many of them offered their sympathy. One in particular said, "It was obvious to all of us that you loved your mother. It was also obvious to all of us that she knew you loved her." Those words were also some of the most comforting and affirming that could have been spoken in such a time of loss and grief. They still come back to me many times and continue to be a source of comfort. I needed to hear the fact that Mom knew we loved her even though it was obvious every time I went to the nursing home. I was always greeted by her wonderful smile. Her smile and the sparkle in her eyes are what I miss the most.

The rest of Monday I spent working on the computer getting the worship aid ready for the funeral. We decided to have Mom's ninetieth birthday picture put on the front because she had that wonderful smile. We also picked out the clothes Mom would wear—the same ones she wore at her ninetieth birthday party. I found my copies of the pictures from the posters and Pat remounted them on foam core boards to put in the back of church before her funeral, and also in the hall where we planned to have the luncheon.

Tuesday was the day to finalize plans and bring the clothes we wanted Mom to wear. Because I had cared so intimately for Mom's physical needs, I asked to dress Mom one last time. I didn't know if Lu, Pat, or Jim would want to help me, but they could choose to do so or not. Jim and Marie flew in mid-morning Tuesday after which we all drove down to Mankato together. We finalized the worship aid and took it to the print shop, then went back to the funeral home to dress Mom. Jim and Pat were not able to help with that task. Lu said she thought she could.

It was the two of us who dressed her so often while she was alive. Pat and Jim never had that privilege because of living so far away.

The funeral director accompanied Lu and me and told us what we could expect. Lu and I slowly and reverently dressed her, and helped the funeral director fix her hair. I cherished every moment I had with her knowing I would never again have the privilege of caring for her body. After we had her all dressed, Pat and Jim came in also. First of all we surrounded her as a family, and then each of us took some alone time with her. It would be our last opportunity. I touched her and kissed her for the last time and I told her how much I loved her and how much I would miss her.

We had not planned a wake on Tuesday evening because so many of Mom's friends were already gone, or not able to come anyway and we were all from out of town. We planned to have a visitation an hour before the funeral Mass in the gathering space at the entry of the church. That way family and friends from out of town did not have to make two trips. They came to see her, visit with us, and attend the funeral. We bought just one spray of flowers for the top of her casket with a rose for each of us with different colors to signify children, grandchildren, and great grandchildren. Roses were her favorite flowers. We set up the posters depicting the different stages of her life, and also had some of her history books around. Many relatives came from out of town, including some of Dad's family. Friends she had in Mankato came, and friends of both Lu and myself. It was a wonderful time to reconnect with family and friends and talk about our memories of who Mom was for all of us. Just before Mass everyone except the immediate family was ushered into the church. The casket was closed and we were given her glasses and her rings. It was a very difficult time. Outside of looking at her pictures, it was the last time we would ever physically see her. This good-bye was the hardest I had ever known.

We involved the family as much as possible in the funeral liturgy. My nephew-in-law, who was a deacon, assisted at Mass and gave the homily. A few of Mom's grandchildren did the readings and the prayers of the faithful. All the rest were pallbearers. Others brought up the wine, water, chalice, and ciborium at the presentation of the gifts. I wanted to give a short eulogy/meditation after communion. Because I was not sure I would be able to do so, I had it all written out and Josie was prepared to read it. Amazingly I was able to do it myself. After the funeral Mass was finished, we proceeded to Calvary Cemetery and buried Mom right next to Dad. The sky was overcast and the temperature was in the 70s. It was pleasant and Mom would have enjoyed being outside.

For Reflection

Mom never spoke directly about dying. When she was still living in her own home, she sometimes referred to the time "when I am gone" as she spoke about who would get her belongings, but it always seemed like something in the very distant future. After her ninetieth birthday, she often asked "Why am I still here?" It seemed more of a rhetorical question than one that she wanted to talk about. For most of Mom's life she did not speak about her feelings. In later years, she was able to verbalize some feelings, but not often, and not in detail. Even though I did ask her sometimes about her feelings, I very rarely met with any success. I was most aware of her feelings by watching her body language, the expressions on her face and the look in her eyes.

As I walked in to see Mom the day before she died, it was the first time she had ever asked who I was. That question was quite unnerving to me. Yet, when she laid her head on my shoulder, it showed me that somewhere deep inside she really did know who I was. She just couldn't give me a name or identify our relationship. When we were outside, and she commented that she couldn't remember anything except what was in front of her, it signified to me that she was living in the present without past or future. I wondered if her inability to look either forward or backward was a way of cushioning the final letting go. Was it a way of preparing her for eternity which is often referred to as an eternal now? I wondered if she would remember her life here or if she would remember me.

Over and over that day she asked me "Why can't I remember anything? What is wrong with me?" Each time she shuddered. I knew she was afraid, but I was not sure what was causing her fear. I sensed she would not be able to tell me if I asked, so I simply gave her my entire presence. It seemed her mind was closing down. Never having experienced it before, I had no idea death was so close. I wonder now if she knew death was so close as I said goodbye to her in the dining room and she asked when she would see

me again. I wonder if she knew and just couldn't
express it.

♦ Did your parent have significant memory loss?

♦ Did your parent always remember who you were? If
not, how did that affect you?

♦ Were you with your parent at death? If not, where
were you and what were your feelings when you
found out?

♦ What was your experience of planning the wake and
funeral? What were your feelings during those days?

♦ What were your highs and lows as you went through
the initial grieving process?

♦ What unanswered questions do you have about
death? About eternal life?

♦ How did your parent's diminishment and death affect
your faith in a loving God?

♦ How do you perceive and feel about your own aging
process?

8 Thin Places

The Celts regarded some places as especially sacred and named them "thin places." These are points of connection and are described as membranes separating the spiritual world from the material world. . . .

Thus, a "thin place" connects the seen and unseen worlds and allows the inhabitants of each world momentarily to cross over to the other. For us, then, it is a place where it is possible to touch and be touched by God as well as the angels, the saints, and those who have died.

John Miriam Jones, S.C.

While family was still surrounding me, I was fine. When the last ones left to go back home, things were very empty and quiet. I was still somewhat in shock and quite numb. I now had time on my hands that I hadn't experienced for years. What was I going to do with this time? I experienced tiredness in both mind and body, yet I did not sleep well at night. Often I woke with the picture in my mind of Mom lying on the bed when I found her, or the day Lu and I had dressed her body for burial. These visions haunted me. Other times I woke picturing Mom at her very sad times, and I felt a pervasive sadness. It was very hard to imagine Mom in eternal life, leaving all this behind her. This was my struggle then, and even though four years have gone by, it is still something with which I grapple, though not as deeply as I did then.

The day after Mom's funeral, I knew I needed to begin my daily exercise routine. As I began my first walk, I recalled finding the walnut after Dad's death, the one that I still carry in my car. As I rounded one of the corners, I noticed a black walnut on the side of the street. It had been run over by a car and was crushed. I had walked this route for five years, and never saw a walnut before. I noticed one of the trees ahead of me and recognized it as a black walnut tree. It was a rather small tree and this was probably the first year it had borne any nuts. Approaching the tree, I noticed a walnut in the tall grass. I bent over to pick it up and found a second joined to it. The symbolism for me was overpowering. Mom and Dad were now together and inseparable. These two walnuts remain on my dresser as a constant reminder that Mom and Dad are still joined as one. This was the first of many signs I had of Mom's presence with me.

The Monday after Mom's funeral, I returned to my work as Pastoral Minister. One of the first calls to come in was from a family at the hospital whose mother had a very severe stroke. We spent the entire afternoon together as they surrounded their mother. She was on life support and they didn't know if she would be able to come back. There was little I could say to them: my ministry was simply to be with them and walk with them through the process. Before the end of the day, a meeting was scheduled the next morning with the doctors, social workers, and chaplain. They asked me to be with them.

The next morning's meeting was extremely difficult as the family was informed that their mother was already, for all purposes, deceased. The only reason she was still alive was because she was attached to the life-support systems. It was an awe-filled experience to be with them as they struggled for hours before making the decision to remove the support systems and let their mother go.

The medical staff asked for a few minutes to remove all the life-support before the family could come back into their mother's room. As they surrounded the bed, her daughter sat close to her head, stroking her cheek. Her husband and I sat next to her. Across from us stood a granddaughter who worked in the medical field. We stood around the bed for the better part of an hour as their mother's breathing, even though not labored, slowed and became very shallow. The sound from the heart monitor had been turned off, so the only sounds in the room were soft weeping and the daughter speaking quietly to her mother. I was watching the mother's neck where I could see her pulse getting weaker and weaker. When it stopped, I also noticed her breathing stopped. I caught the eye of the granddaughter and mouthed "Grandma is gone." She checked her grandmother's pulse and then informed the rest of the family. The daughter broke into sobs and said her final good-byes. I stayed with the family until they left the hospital. We prayed together at different times. Since another part of my ministry was to help people plan and arrange the funeral liturgy, I accompanied the family through the funeral and burial.

Reflecting on my experience with this family, I can't imagine how I was able to be totally present to them through this entire experience, since I myself was in such deep grief over the loss of my own mother. I went home both days feeling like a limp dishrag, and just sat in the living room in numbness, without any perceptive thoughts. However, I may have done the same had I not been asked to walk with them. At some point in time I realized how grateful I was that my family never had to make that kind of a life and death decision for Mom.

After Mom had moved to the nursing home, another woman whom I have known for many years moved into her apartment. Carol came to tell me something that had happened to her the week after Mom died. One afternoon when she returned home from shopping, she could not find her checkbook. She called the store, searched her car, searched the apartment, and turned her purse inside out without finding it. She was worried sick. The next morning she went to the bank to stop payment on her checks. She said she prayed before she left, "Hilda, you lived here for a while, you probably know where I put my checkbook. Please help me find it." After arriving at the bank, she told her story to one of the bank employees. While the employee walked away momentarily to get some information, Carol opened her purse and found her checkbook right on the top. She confidently attributed the discovery to Mom's intervention.

About two weeks after Mom's death I came home after work and found my sister-in-law, Dottie's, telephone number on the caller ID, but there was no message. When I returned her call she told me that she had been in bed sick for three days and had not used the phone. She asked her husband, Rolie, who said he had not called either. I could not figure it out. Suddenly thoughts came together for me. Mom and Dad had grieved deeply when my brother, Bob, Dottie's first husband, died of cancer at age forty-eight. They struggled when Dottie remarried about a year after he died. Mom especially was not able to accept Dottie's second marriage. There was no earthly explanation for the number on the caller ID. It occurred to me that finally Mom was able to forgive Dottie and was now letting me know. I wondered if forgiveness and reconciliation are possible even after death? I can't help wondering if Mom is also with Bob and my other two brothers who died as infants.

One Sunday morning at Mass, I felt Mom next to me. At first she was ninety-two, the age at her death. Then, suddenly, she was the young woman whose picture sat on my piano. I became conscious of Dad on the other side of me, at first as the seventy-eight-year-old he was when he died, and then as a young man. Often when I visited them on weekends, I sat between them when we went to Sunday Mass. Here I was experiencing that again, but in a way that was so new and different. Their presence was only momentary and brought tears to my eyes. It opened up all kinds of questions about life after death, and about how those who die experience eternal life. Many times I spoke with Mom and asked questions. "Who are you now since you are no longer the little old lady I took care of for such a long time? Would it be possible to know you as the young woman who had so many friends? Will I ever be able to know you in the fullness of who you were/are? Can relationships continue to deepen after one person has died? Can we come to know each other in a new way not possible while both of us were alive?"

Three weeks after Mom's death, I spent a weekend on the north shore of Lake Superior. The weather was absolutely fabulous. Josie had gone to Duluth mid-week for a conference that ended Friday afternoon and I planned to leave at noon Friday to meet her there. As I drove out of the garage, I was thinking how Mom and Dad loved to travel and so I invited them to come along knowing how they loved the scenery around Lake Superior. I turned on the car radio and the first words I heard were "Soft as the voice of an angel..." from Mom's favorite song, "Whispering Hope." It brought back childhood memories and reminded me of the times I played "Name That Tune" with Mom in the nursing home. When she couldn't think of the song title, she was able to sing those words of the first line. Whispering Hope. is just not a song that is played on the stations I usually listen to on the radio. It didn't really matter what station it was on because to me it was just another way for Mom to let me know she was with me. I wondered if these kinds of experiences are simply coincidence or if they are a new kind of consciousness?

At the very end of that month, I was still writing thank-you notes to people who had sent cards and/or memorials. I had received an azalea plant from Growing Through Loss, a grief coalition with which I worked in the Twin Cities area. One morning as I sat by the dining room table, I glanced at the azalea and noticed it was so wilted because I forgot to water it. I knew from experience that the entire plant could die. It was a memorial for Mom and I was devastated. I began to cry. Quickly I watered it, all the while praying to Mom. I reminded her that I had not had a visible sign of her presence for over a week. Could she please help restore the azalea plant? I left the house for the day, and when I returned late in the afternoon the blossoms were all fresh and vibrant as they had been the previous day. I looked at Mom's picture on the piano and caught that sparkle in her eye. She again let me know she was with me.

The times I felt Mom's presence were very comforting to me. However, the times between seemed very long and lonely. My parish ministry kept me busy all week. When there were no evening meetings, I often just sat quietly in the living room. I couldn't stand listening to TV or even music. I just needed to "zone out," feeling exhausted and having no physical or psychological energy to do anything. This was time to just be and try to heal the big empty hole in my heart. On the weekends it was very hard to get going to do anything except what was essential for day-to-day living. It seemed important to get as much physical exercise as possible by walking on a daily basis and taking long bike rides on the weekends. The lack of energy did not dissolve quickly. It was impossible to change my lifestyle overnight after years of caring for Mom. I realize now how very important this kind of self-care was in my grief process.

Grief has a way of piling up, and in the grief coalition we refer to that as the "domino effect." I am not sure I really grieved sufficiently after Dad's death because I was so concerned about Mom. Yes, there were some times I grieved, but I put a lot of my grief on the back burner. In grieving the loss of Mom, a lot of it was done before she died as I dealt with her diminishment. After she died, much of the grief I experienced was also for Dad. Slowly, over time the grief has given way to gratitude for who each of them were for me through the years. I so want to be able to see them again and know them as they are now.

During my time of grief, I would often journal about my feelings, questions, and experiences of Mom's presence. It was only after writing pages and pages of memories that the thought of doing this book was born. Ministry at the parish kept me very busy with little time to do other than continue to journal during my times of prayer.

In June, the summer after Mom's death, I made a retreat at the Christian Brother's retreat center in Dunrovin. There had been a mix-up in the scheduling, and Josie and I were not able to stay in the little cabin we had originally reserved. Instead we were given the guesthouse that was already occupied by the new director and his family. Jerome and Mary had three young daughters and had moved into the house just the week before. They were willing to move out for the week and let us use the space. When we met them, Mary told us that the name Josie was very special because they gave the name Josie to their little girl who died before birth. Mary said I looked so familiar to her. As we continued to talk and I told her about Mom's death the previous summer, Mary made the connection and asked if my mom was Hilda. Mary had worked at the nursing home and cared for Mom. She recalled Mom's sense of humor. She also mentioned that she observed the good care we gave Mom. This conversation with Mary was another affirmation for me to seriously consider writing a book in order to tell my story.

During that same retreat, I was sitting outside reading and reflecting and Josie was sitting at some distance from me. All of a sudden she cried, "Ouch!" It was then I discovered the tree under which we were sitting was a huge black walnut tree. The wind had knocked a walnut off and it fell on top of Josie's head. As we laughed, I felt Mom there and could almost hear her laughing with us. In fact I even wondered if she had anything to do with the falling of the nut to get our attention to her presence, especially since the seeds of this book were sprouting.

Last year I called the doctor's office to set up an eye appointment. The receptionist asked my name and how to spell it, then promptly asked if my mother was Hilda

Friesen. She identified herself as one of the aides who had worked with Mom at the nursing home. She, too, remembered Mom fondly and commented on how our family took such good care of her. Mom had been in the nursing home for only a short time, yet it seems she made an impression on many of those who worked with her.

Since it has been almost four years since Mom's death, my thoughts turn often to the pleasant memories. I am filled with gratitude for Mom and for the time I was able to care for her and grow close to her in a way that would never otherwise have happened. At the eulogy for her funeral I answered for myself the question she asked so often, "Why am I still here?" My answer remains the same today. "Mom, it's so I could learn to love you more deeply."

For Reflection

There are other memories that come back to me but I have expressed the most poignant ones here. These are my "thin places" where I have been touched by God and by Mom. They bring me comfort and a confidence in the faith I proclaim.

♦ Have you experienced "thin places" ? In other words, times, events or places that allow the seen and unseen places to connect?

♦ How have they affected your relationship with your parent and with God?

♦ If you can recall no "thin places," how has the absence of your parent called you to grow both personally and spiritually?

9 My Memory Journey

Nothing can make up for the absence of
someone whom we love. . . .
It is nonsense to say that God fills the gap;
God doesn't fill it,
but on the contrary, God keeps it empty
and so helps us to keep alive our former
communion with each other, even at the
cost of pain. . . .
The dearer and richer our memories, the
more difficult the separation.
But gratitude changes the pangs of memory
into tranquil joy.
The beauties of the past are borne, not as a
thorn in the flesh, but as a precious
gift in themselves.

Dietrich Bonhoeffer

Often I thought about how Mom and Dad loved
to travel, and how they had once taken me back
to where both of them grew up. One thing Mom never
forgot was the fact she was born in Victoria, Kansas. In
her story she had told me how her Dad had worked on
the Union Pacific Railroad and they moved from town to
town as he helped to maintain the tracks. I decided I
wanted to take a memory journey back to Kansas during

the summer of 1999. It just seemed this would be a way of continuing to do my grief work, and also be a wonderful tribute to Mom's love of visiting with family. There are no close relatives living in Victoria, and only a few of my cousins living in various other cities in Kansas. Mom's sisters had moved to Denver, Colorado, where most of their children still live. I wanted to see as many as possible so I called ahead and made arrangements. I also asked Mom to accompany me so I could experience the wonderful history of her childhood and family.

Josie consented to go with me, and we gave ourselves three weeks. The first town in which we stopped was Gorham, Kansas. One of Mom's favorite cousins had lived there when I was growing up. As we spoke to different people, no one had any recollection of the family. When we visited the church we ran into the Sister who was the Pastoral Minister. As it was mid-afternoon, I asked her if there was a motel in Victoria where we could stay for the night. She informed us that Victoria was much too small a town to have a motel, but she had heard there was a bed and breakfast we might want to look for.

Long before we got to Victoria, we could see the two spires of St. Fidelis Church. Mom had often talked about watching the farmers build the church when she was a child. She was born in 1906 and the church was finished in 1912. Because of its size, it was dubbed the Cathedral of the Plains. She also talked about the Capuchin priests who worked at the parish and the St. Agnes Sisters who taught in the school. Mom's aunt, my great-aunt, had entered the St. Agnes Sisters whose motherhouse is in Fond du Lac, Wisconsin. As we drove down the short main street we looked for signs for a bed and breakfast. Not finding it, we finally stopped to ask a teenage boy if he knew where it was. He informed us there was a bed and breakfast but he wanted us to talk to his mother. She came out of the house and told us she would get in her car and lead us there.

Since it was almost suppertime when we arrived at the bed and breakfast, we inquired about a restaurant from the couple who owned it. The restaurant was across the railroad tracks. Mention of the tracks reminded me that Mom said the town was split into the German and English sectors when she was growing up. Crossing the tracks meant we were leaving the original Herzog or German sector and entering the original Victoria or English sector. While at the restaurant, the owner came over to talk to us, knowing we were not from the area. I told her who I was and why we were there. She recognized my Mom's maiden name of Weigel and wondered if she was related to me. She disappeared and came back with a genealogy done by the parish, and found out we were shirttail relatives. We had a very pleasant exchange. She gave me the book to take for the evening and asked me to return it to her the next morning.

After supper, instead of going back to the bed and breakfast right away, we went to the church to see if we could get inside to see it. Since it was already locked for the night, we walked the streets surrounding the church. The original St. Joseph's school that Mom had attended through eighth grade was gone, but the cornerstone was preserved in the new school that was built on the same spot. A woman who lived across the street saw us and came over to talk. She was a lifetime member of the parish and gave us a lot of history. We talked for almost two hours. She told us there was an 8 a.m. Mass the next morning, and we could get history books from the church office afterward.

Since it was still light when we finished our conversation we went to the cemetery that we had passed on our way into town. As I walked the rows of markers, many names were familiar to me because Mom had talked about them. Our family also had a genealogy done by one of Mom's cousins, in which many of those names were recorded. We were there just at sunset and Kansas gave us a spectacular show of color as the sun went down over the wheat fields.

We returned to the bed and breakfast and spent an enjoyable evening with the couple who owned it. They had a huge house and gave us a suite of rooms we could have all to ourselves. As we visited that evening, we looked through the book we had borrowed from the restaurant owner, and also found this couple to be distant relatives of mine. We spent the evening tracing our relationship, and swapping family stories.

The next morning we got up in time to go to the church for Mass. One of the ladies who worked at the parish left the church lights on after Mass so I could get pictures of the inside. I also took pictures of the statues across the street, a memorial to the Volga Germans who arrived in Victoria April 6, 1876. We went over to the office, looked at all the history books they had, and purchased what I wanted. Every once in a while I take time to go through the books again. When we returned to the bed and breakfast the couple had a wonderful brunch for us. After packing up our things we returned the book borrowed from the restaurant owner and moved on. I left Victoria with warm feelings because of the wonderful hospitality we received from Mom's people.

Mom had talked about Emmeram and Catharine, Kansas. She spoke mainly of the churches she attended in each of these places. We located Emmeram on the map, but could not find it so we had to ask two different farmers how to get there. We were very surprised to find out there was no town, but only the church. It had burned two years before our trip, after having been abandoned for many years. The stone walls were still standing, but everything else had been destroyed. It was surrounded by wheat fields and very hard to see from any distance. Catharine was easy to find and was a very small town. I stopped only long enough to get pictures of the church. I knew no one would be familiar with my family.

The next place we visited was Hays. After Mom's mother had surgery at the hospital in Hays, Mom had to live and work at the hospital to pay off the bill. We were not able to find the hospital, but we did find St. Joseph's Church which I figured Mom attended while she lived in Hays. As we drove around the city we found the studio of the artist who made the figures of the memorial in Victoria. He had a huge statue of a St. Agnes Sister in the yard. We took time to visit with him and see his entire studio. A few blocks away there was another memorial to the Volga Germans—a model of the type of homes they built with the local stone. I was experiencing my Mom's history.

There were a couple other small towns Mom had mentioned, Ellis and Quinter, but when we got there neither one seemed to hold the history comparable to what we had already found. We moved on to WaKeeney and stayed overnight with one of my cousins, Carolyn. Her mom, my Aunt Minnie (Wilhelmina), had died when she was very young, and Carolyn lived with us for a while because Mom had promised Minnie she would take care of Carolyn after her death. However, a family heard about Carolyn from my Uncle Aquiline, who still lived in Kansas at that time. Because they could not have any children of their own the man came to Mom in Mankato and begged to adopt Carolyn.

I was about six years old when he came and I still remember him as a very tall man. Mom did not want to let Carolyn go, but when she asked the opinion of her siblings, they agreed to let the man and his wife adopt Carolyn. When all the legal paperwork was completed, Carolyn went back to WaKeeney, Kansas, to live with him and his wife.

The conversations with Carolyn were filled with wonderful stories from our family history and our time was all too short. Garden City was the next stop where we visited with a couple more of my cousins, Rose and Louise, daughters of my aunt Blanche. Here, again, we swapped some wonderful family history. During the conversation I found out that Rose had cancer and the situation did not look good. I am so glad I went when I did so I could talk to her. Rose died less than a year after I was there.

All the rest of the relatives I planned to visit were in and around Denver. Most of them were the children of my Mom's youngest sister, Aunt Rose, and many of them are younger than myself. We stayed at Theresa's house, arriving there Friday evening. We had planned to be there on the weekend when people were not working, and it gave us the best opportunity to see them. Theresa had planned to have everyone over for Saturday afternoon, early supper. She is the one in the family with all the German recipes and Saturday Josie and I had a chance to help Theresa and her sisters with the meal preparation. After a brief lunch, my cousin Mena took us to the cemetery where Grandma and Grandpa (Mom's parents) are buried. We also visited Aunt Minnie's grave, which is in the same cemetery. By the time we arrived back at Theresa's, most of the family had already arrived. We began to share stories and pictures. The entire evening was a delightful experience, full of good conversation and much laughter. Again, the time was all too short. Long before we wanted it to end, the time came for everyone to leave.

Sunday morning Josie and I attended Mass at a nearby church. I was surprised by the name of the priest, Father Hall, and stopped to visit with him after Mass because his name was familiar. Helen Hall is Mom's cousin who had compiled our family genealogy. I discovered that Helen was Father Hall's aunt. He told me that Helen had died a couple of years earlier, which explained why a letter I sent to her came back to me.

Sunday afternoon Theresa and her husband had another engagement, so it gave me time to visit with Mena. A couple years earlier I had been in Colorado Springs for a conference and visited Mena and her mother, Aunt Rose. Since then Aunt Rose had died and Mena was moving to Denver. We had been in communication since the visit and thoroughly enjoyed having this much time together. Mena had to leave for home, a small town to the east of Denver, after supper. Josie and I stayed at Theresa's one more night and left early the next morning.

We moved on to visit some other family and friends before returning home. My memory journey was finished. It was a wonderful experience! I have looked at the photos many times and remembered all my experiences with family. Somehow I know Mom was with me during that time because I felt her presence. I'm sure she was very pleased that I cherished her wonderful memories enough to go back and try to imagine her in all the places where she grew up. For me, this trip was a time to process some of my grief, to continue healing and discover even more who my Mom was and continues to be for me. I was able to move on to a deeper gratitude for her, her family, her life and mine.

There were many times I clashed with my mom, especially when I was a teenager. Earlier in my life, I am not so sure I ever really wanted to be like her. During the time I was caring for her, I didn't have time to reflect on that possibility. One experience on my memory journey pulled me into thinking about this reality. When I rang my cousin Rose's doorbell, her first words to me when she answered the door were, "Here is Hilda all over again!" Josie told me that I was like Mom in many ways. I have since spent time reflecting on how that is so. Not only do I have physical characteristics like Mom, such as my hands, but there are other character traits as well. Many people have said they loved Mom because she listened to them. My ministry in parishes as a Pastoral Minister is primarily a listening presence for those who are in pain. I know I am a compassionate listener because of the way people so often relax in my presence and openly tell me their stories.

For Reflection

As a member of a religious community, I have no children of my own who will continue to bear Mom's physical and character traits. I have to be satisfied that my sisters and brothers will hand them on through their children. But it is a comfort to know that Mom still lives on in me. Perhaps I have handed on the gift of listening to all those I have trained as ministers of listening in my professional work.

♦ Is there a journey you need to take to help you move through the grieving process?

♦ Perhaps a trip to your childhood home and neighborhood, or getting in touch with relatives?

♦ Would it help to write down the story of your parents' life, or gather pictures into an album? Maybe your journey will be through memories as you move toward wholeness and gratitude.

♦ In what ways are you like your parent(s)? What gifts or traits did you get from them?

♦ Are you grateful for these?

♦ Are there gifts or traits you would rather not have inherited?

♦ How does your parent(s) live on in you?

Afterword

I give You thanks, O Blessed One,
With all my heart; before all the people
I sing your praise. . . .
You are a very Presence as I face my
fears and doubts;
Your strength upholds me.

Nan C. Merrill

With deep gratitude and thanks, I bring this book
to its close. You have read my story and heard the
questions that caring for my mom brought to me. Writing
this book has been a meaningful way to process my grief
as I continue to walk my faith journey. My hope for you,
the reader, is that you will give yourself time to grieve
and to wrestle with the questions that arise from your
own experience of care giving.

As you grieve, may you continue to probe the mystery
of who your parent was and continues to be for you. May
your gratitude grow deeper with each memory. And may
that love and gratitude propel you outward to care
compassionately for others.

I gratefully acknowledge all who have played a key role in helping this book become a reality. My first and deepest thanks goes to the members of my family with whom I walked during the fourteen years I cared for Mom. My sister, Luella Bellomo, shared the weight of Mom's care. From a distance my other siblings, Jim Friesen and Pat French, remained in regular communication with both of us and readily supported the many decisions we made. I thank each one of them from the bottom of my heart.

Secondly, I want to thank the members of my religious community who supported and sustained me. On a daily basis, Josetta Marie Spencer, SSND, shared my experiences, frustrations, questions, and doubts. She not only provided support through the initial ideas of writing this book, but she proofread every word of it. Likewise, I am indebted to the leadership of the Mankato Province of the School Sisters of Notre Dame who gave me the gift of several months to write this book and the emotional, psychological and financial support to bring it to completion. In particular, I am grateful to my SSND mentors and friends who assisted by reading the manuscript, making corrections and suggestions: Inez Hoey, SSND; Carmen Madigan, SSND; and Joseph Marie Kasel, SSND.

I give special acknowledgment to Ave Maria Press for its vision in providing printed resources to those who minister to the bereaved and especially to Eileen M. Ponder, my editor, for her professional expertise. There are many others, too numerous to mention here, to whom I extend my gratitude for their contribution to this endeavor, especially my colleagues in ministry and the aides who shared the day-to-day care for Mom during the last year-and-a-half of her life. For all of these, I am profoundly grateful.

Beatitudes for Friends of the Aged

Blessed are they who understand
my faltering step and palsied hand.

Blessed are they who know that my ears today
must strain to catch the things they say.

Blessed are they who seem to know
that my eyes are dim and my wits are slow.

Blessed are they who looked away
when coffee spilled at table today.

Blessed are they with a cheery smile
who stop to chat for a little while.

Blessed are they who never say,
"You've told that story twice today."

Blessed are they who know the ways
to bring back memories of yesterdays.

Blessed are they who make it known
that I'm loved, respected and not alone.

Blessed are they who know I'm at a loss
to find the strength to carry the Cross.

Blessed are they who ease the days
on my journey Home in loving ways.

Esther Mary Walker

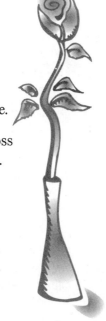

Resources

For Caregivers

Bartocci, Barbara. *Nobody's Child Anymore: Grieving, Caring, and Comforting When Parents Die*. Sorin Books, 2000.

Edenberg, Mark A. *Talking with Your Aging Parents*. Shambhala Publications, 1987.

Farr, Mary I. *If I Could Mend Your Heart*. Book Peddlers, 2001.

Greenberg, Vivian. *Children of a Certain Age: Becoming Friends with Your Aging Parents*. Macmillan, Inc., Lexington Books, 1994.

Lewis, C. S. *A Grief Observed*. Seabury Press, 1963.

Nouwen, Henri J.M. *A Letter of Consolation*. Harper Collins, 1982.

Samples, Larson, and Larson. *Self-Care for Caregivers: A Twelve Step Approach*. Hazelden, 1991.

Schiff, Harriet Sarnoff. *How Did I Become My Parent's Parent?* Viking Press, 1996.

Silverstone, Barbara and Helen Kandal Hyman. *You and Your Aging Parent*. Pantheon Books, 1976.

Starkman, Elaine Marcus. *Learning to Sit in the Silence: A Journal of Caretaking*. Papier Mache Press, 1993.

Westburg, Granger. *Good Grief*. Fortress Press, 1962.

For Those Embracing Life's Later Years

Berman, Philip, ed. *The Courage to Grow Old*. Ballantine, 1989.

Fischer, Kathleen. *Winter Grace: Spirituality and Aging*. Upper Room Books, 1998.

Fischer, Kathleen. *Autumn Gospel: Women in the Second Half of Life*. Paulist Press, 1995.

Hinton, Pat Corrick. *Time to Become Myself: Reflections on Growing Older*. CompCare, 1990.

Morgan, Richard L. *Remembering Your Story: A Guide to Spiritual Autobiography*. The Upper Room, 1996.

Nouwen, Henri J.M. and Walter J. Gaffney. *Aging: The Fulfillment of Life*. A Doubleday Image Book, 1976.

Saussy, Carroll. *The Art of Growing Old: A Guide to Faithful Aging*. Augsburg, 1998.

Thibault, Jane Marie. *A Deepening Love Affair: The Gift of God in Later Life*. The Upper Room, 1993.

Wicks, Robert J. *After 50: Spiritually Embracing Your Own Wisdom Years*. Paulist Press, 1997.

Wiederkehr, Macrina. *Gold in Your Memories: Sacred Moments, Glimpses of God*. Ave Maria Press, 2000.

LYNETTE FRIESEN, SSND, has served the Archdiocese of St. Paul/ Minneapolis for over thirty years in a variety of educational and pastoral settings. She holds a master's degree in theology with a concentration in pastoral ministry from Seattle University and a certificate in pastoral leadership from St. Paul Seminary, School of Divinity at the University of St. Thomas.

With the support of her family, close friends, and community, she cared for her aging mother for the last fourteen years of her mother's life.